THE FLOAT
TANK CURE

FREE YOURSELF FROM STRESS, ANXIETY, AND PAIN THE NATURAL WAY

by
SHANE STOTT

Published by Shane Stott

Printed by DiggyPOD
Tecumseh, MI
www.diggypod.com

For ordering information or special discounts for bulk purchases, contact Shane Stott at thefloattankcure@gmail.com

Edited by: Amy Anderson (andersoncontent.com)
Layout and Page Design by: Jason Malaska
Cover design by: Ralph N. and Jeff Holmes
Online Content Creation by: Jaymie Tarshis (jaymietarshis.com)

ISBN: 978-0-9966257-0-8

Printed in the United States of America on acid-free paper

First Edition

CONTENTS

FORWARD

I first floated in my basement in a float tank that was Frankenstein's monster, built from a farming fertilizer tank and a collection of aquarium parts. My friends thought I was building an over sized water coffin, but it was the opposite. My life was a fragile mess, my mind a constant static louder than channel 72 after a late night infomercial, and I needed solace.

That night, I found it.

Floating in that dark tank, suspended by lukewarm salt water, I felt like I was floating in orbit, untouched by gravity. The silence was visceral, and the effect profound.

My journey from then to now being owner of a float tank manufacturing company has been a long one. Sometimes lonely, sometimes scary. And it's why I do what I do. I want to share the power of the float with anybody out there who like me is looking for solace. For silence. For more meaning. For a deeper connection. This book is for you. It's meant to be your guide as you make the journey, and the discovery that I did.

Happy Floating,

-Shane Stott

This book is dedicated to adversity.
Thanks for the great story.

HE WHO KNOWS
HIMSELF IS
ENLIGHTENED.
-LAO TZU

INTRODUCTION

'm Shane Stott, and I'm grateful to say that today my life is pretty damn good. I live in Utah. I'm married to an incredible woman named Jamie. We are the proud parents to a baby boy named Grayson and a couple of fur babies, Weezy and Indy. Life has turned out really nice for me.

Especially given the fact that about ten years ago I wasn't sure I was going to keep living it.

At the time I was in a huge battle in Los Angeles, far away from where I had grown up in Utah. Don't get me wrong: The battle was in my head.

It was 2005 and I was in trade school for music production. I had a dream of becoming a record producer. School, networking, my job—it was all stressful. I worked long hours and many weekends, sometimes spending all day in the recording studio. I would trade a good night's sleep for a head start on a project. I would trade a day of enjoyment and relaxation for a chance at a new opportunity. I was cutting out all the pieces of a balanced life in exchange for a dream. I didn't realize it yet, but I was selling my happiness and well-being for what I thought was success.

What's funny about the onset of a mental disorder is that everything can seem to be going just "fine." It's like living two lives—you can take the good view or you can look at the reality underneath.

Good view: I was graduating school in Los Angeles and working on a great career in the music industry. I was paying my dues and earning my stripes by working long hours and learning my craft. I had a job in the recording industry, and I was meeting great people to advance my career.

Reality: I was in a new place with no family or close friends for support. I was in a broken long distance relationship, and because I was stubborn, I wasn't reaching out to anybody for help. The long days, nights, and weekends were catching up to me, and my anxieties were growing to unmanageable levels. I was drinking after the long days in an effort to force myself into relaxation. It would work for the night, but the next morning my mental state would be worse.

Each day I worked hard and forgot about my fears for a few hours, only to repeat the process that night. Behind closed doors, I was falling into a dark place. The people I worked with were empathetic, and my girlfriend eventually moved out to Los Angeles to live with me. But secretly I felt all alone.

"I WAS SELLING MY HAPPINESS AND WELL-BEING FOR WHAT I THOUGHT WAS SUCCESS."

I was constantly thinking, "I don't feel good, I feel sad, I feel stressed, I'm not sure how long I can do this," but I would put some event or goal just out of reach so I was forced to keep running for happiness. I just needed to get my girlfriend out to live with me, finish this project, make a little more money, get some more sleep, and on and on. The truth is nothing I could do, achieve, or accomplish was going to fix the way I felt inside. I was sprinting through a marathon race. I was searching for happiness and life fulfillment outside of me.

THE BREAK

In the fall of 2005, my company attended a trade show in Las Vegas. We had prepared for weeks prior to the trip. The plan was to work our booth and get more clients into our recording company. I was in charge of building the booth and had spent the week leading up to departure working 16-hour days. Before the show I pulled an all-nighter and then drove to Vegas with the crew.

The pressure and lack of sleep added to my already spiraling anxiety. I was like a thread pulled so taught I could feel myself fraying.

Once in Vegas, we got everything set up thanks to a constant stream of energy drinks and coffee, and somehow I made it through the first day. That night we decided to celebrate. Oh how I wish we would have celebrated by getting some sleep! Instead, I drank all night and don't remember much of anything. I don't know how, but the next day, we got up and worked the second day of the show fueled by more energy drinks and coffee. But this time, something was different.

I felt tremors run through my body. My eyelids constantly twitched. I was scared by the symptoms, but I kept moving.

Later that night at dinner as we sat around the table, someone mentioned that I had seemed pretty out of it since the night before. Like a zombie. Like I wasn't even there.

But I was there. Only I felt like I was in a constant state of fear and that my world was barely held together in my mind. After dinner I went back to my room and got in bed to try and calm down. *What is wrong with me? Why do I feel this impending sense of doom like my life is going to collapse?* I felt like I was going crazy, and the thought crushed me. My heart sank.

My uncle had been diagnosed with schizophrenia when he was eighteen years old. His whole life collapsed into a mess. Our entire family was affected, and I grew up hearing and seeing the pain it caused. Even as a kid, I worried that this kind of mental collapse could happen to me.

As my anxiety incapacitated me and fear overtook me in that hotel room, I became convinced I was headed down the same road as my uncle. I was terrified of my own mind and what I saw as a bleak future filled with heartache for everyone I loved.

The terror of going crazy threw my mind and body into a physical state of panic. My chest sank in, I began to sweat, and I couldn't breathe. *What is going on?* As my body verified my fears that I was going crazy, I spun out over the edge of self-control, and it felt like something inside me broke.

I panted in that tiny room, playing out scenes of what might happen next. I felt the stab of embarrassment and shame at the idea of paramedics coming to my room to get me, being admitted to a mental ward, losing my girlfriend, my friends, my family. Dread at never being the same again overtook me like a whirlwind. I shook at the weight of my thoughts. I tried to breathe.

Stumbling to the bathroom, I turned on the water in the tub. I stripped and lay down, sinking my ears under the rising water. The thunder of the tap filling the tub and thrum of my heartbeat slowed the churning of my thoughts. The water soothed my clenched muscles. I stayed there for an hour, floating in a warm cocoon, until my breathing returned to normal.

Afterwards, I crawled into bed and managed to fall asleep, hoping that whatever had just happened would never happen again.

THE DESCENT

If you've had anxiety, you know what a downward spiral it is. The battle of anxiety quickly turns into a battle with depression because you just can't figure out how to be happy when you're constantly afraid. The depression keeps you from living your life to the fullest, meeting your obligations, having relationships. Which all serves to create more anxiety and panic.

The next morning when I woke in my hotel room, my first feeling was fear as I wondered, *Is it still there?*

It was. And the fear of the panic returning actually escalated my anxiety to yet another state of panic. Like a wave, it overtook me.

I remember trying to keep it together when I got home after the trip. I clung to my girlfriend, and for a brief time I felt okay. The problem was I was clinging to her for my safety. I was no doubt smothering her, and within weeks she was gone. Once she was gone, I went into an even darker hole. A hole of isolation.

Isolation feels good when you're struggling with depression and anxiety because you don't have to deal with anyone. It allows you to be yourself with no expectations. The danger is that you're not talking through your issues with others. There is so much benefit to talking with friends and family. It allows you to hear your problems out loud so you can measure how serious they really are or not. A third party is necessary because no matter how much you've thought through your problems, it's still you doing the thinking. You have blind spots that only others can point out.

But I didn't ask anyone else for help or input. I didn't talk about the hell I was living. And for the next few months, I was caught in an evil loop of dread that the panic would return—and that dread itself triggered the attacks.

At the end, my mental state was so bad, a caffeinated drink would send me into a panic tail spin. I was so nerved up that my vision would actually shake, and I would have to close my eyes to make it stop. I was on edge all day until about midnight when my mind would crash from exhaustion. The second I woke up, I instantly wondered again and again, *Is it still there?* And as sure as the sunrise, it was.

THE HOPE

I was totally in the dark about why I was suffering so much back then. What I know today is that I didn't arrive at anxiety by chance. I realize now that a mix of isolation, alcohol, trying times, and a very sensitive nervous system proved to be dangerous for me.

When I could no longer stand my existence in Los Angeles and my career began to derail, I flat out collapsed my life and had to start from scratch. I moved back home with my family and finally saw a psychiatrist, who prescribed me anti-panic and anti-depressant medications. I had sessions with a string of counselors to help me learn how to think and process, balance and relax. I had to learn how to cope in an overloaded world with a sensitive nervous system. The medication and the therapy began to give me hope that maybe I could lead a normal life, but I still found day-to-day tasks a struggle.

Sometime in my journey back to a healthy brain in 2007, I discovered an amazing tool to achieve peace and happiness: meditation.

Many people hear meditation and think "Oh yeah,

I know about that and it never worked for me." They dismiss everything else that is said about it.

I'd like to ask you a favor. While you read this book, pretend that meditation is something you've never heard of before. In fact, as soon as you come across a term or an idea or a practice in this book that makes your mind snap shut and dismiss it as useless, ineffective, or not applicable to your circumstance, pretend you've never heard of it. Try reading with an open mind what I and others in this book have to say to you. That's what I had to do when I first started learning about meditation, and it has altered the entire course of my life.

The meditation that happens in a float tank is something much deeper and more profound than any meditation that can be done outside of the tank. And we'll talk more about that in later chapters. But let me talk to you about the first steps of meditation and the impact it had on my profound mental disorder.

"THEREISNOTHINGMOREPOWERFULTHAN PURE, FOCUSED ATTENTION."

My therapist was the first to challenge me to try meditating. Even if it was just guided meditation on iTunes. At the time I was willing to try just about anything because I needed more relief than I could get from prescription medication alone. Using guided meditation recordings made it very easy to do. I just threw on my headphones at night and let folks like Karin Leonard take me on a guided hippie journey through what looked—in my imagination—like the forests of

Avatar. (Don't ask me why but when I get to envision my own forest it always looks like an over-the-top Disney movie. Don't judge me.)

Guided meditations are so easy. For those of you not familiar, these are meditations where you hear nature sounds or calming music while someone speaks to you and leads you through of a series of imagined scenarios all intended to relax you or bring you to a place of peace. Frankly, I don't understand why they're not more popular.*

After about a week of guided mediations each night, I knew I had found another element in what I referred to as "my calm life strategy."

Meditation not only helps me to become calm in the moment, but its effects are lasting throughout my day. Almost like my life is a giant projection of my inner state.

While guided meditation is awesome, I soon discovered that real, "mind-off" meditation isn't so easy.

Have you ever tried to *not* think about something? It's basically impossible. Let me show you: Do not think of a pink elephant. Did you just see a giant Pepto-Bismol colored Dumbo?

Exactly.

It's the same with not thinking. You tell yourself not to think and you realize that's a thought. It never ends. In fact the best way I've found to not think is to count backwards from one hundred to zero, breathing in and out with every number and watching the numbers in my mind.

*Email me and I'll send you links to my favorite guided meditations thefloattankcure@gmail.com

If I ever start thinking of anything else, I just bring myself back to the counting and start back at one hundred. It's a tad challenging but it works.

If you can master the thoughts, you are about halfway there.

The other half is dealing with distractions. Whether it's a dog barking, a car driving by, or a text message, distractions are constant. Okay, so let's say you lock yourself in a room with no cell phone and you're in the middle of nowhere. Great! No distractions, right? You should be meditating perfectly in no time, right? Wrong. Now you've got your body to distract you. Have you ever sat or lay down for a long time in one position? Next thing you know you need to move. Maybe your leg falls asleep or your pillow needs adjusting. Whatever it is, it's a distraction, and it makes pure meditation very, very tricky.

So I practiced. (Yes, that's why they call it meditation practice. It takes a lot of it.) And once I started seeing results, I realized that there is nothing more powerful than pure, focused attention. The times when I reached this state were unreal, almost like I was experiencing my authentic self, which is a state and feeling, *not* thoughts.

Thoughts were the damn things that got me into all the trouble in the first place. If there's one thing I've learned through battles with anxiety it's that I'm the observer of my thoughts and my thoughts are not me.

THE CURE

Filled with even more hope for a normal, peaceful life—maybe even one without medication—I started searching for better ways to meditate. Outside of a softer pillow and quieter room, I couldn't think of much. Then I watched a video.

I was up late one night browsing easier ways to meditate, and I remember stumbling onto a device called an isolation tank. (It's also called a float tank, a sensory deprivation tank, an isolation chamber, or a mix of those keywords.) I remember thinking these tanks were kind of freaky but how cool was the idea of shutting the world off? Then I watched a video of a guy named Joe Rogan, who at the time was the host of the TV show *Fear Factor*. He was into floating, so I thought, It must be *somewhat* legit.

In fact, Joe had a podcast where he talked frequently about float tanks. Someone had compiled his best sound clips, thrown up some graphics, and made a video that I watched over and over.

It. Was. Killer.

This video* inspired me like I had never been inspired before. I *had* to have one of these tanks. I knew how hard pure meditation could be for a high strung person like myself, and I knew how great it made me feel. Now I had discovered there was a machine that could make it easy. I was sold.

Without taking you through the details just yet, I ended up building a float tank in my basement from scratch using mostly materials you could buy at Home

*Want to see the video? Check out
TheFloatTankCure.com

22

Depot.

From that day on, I've had my own float tank right here at home—my own meditation machine.

"FLOATING SHOULD BE A STAPLE FOR ANYONE SEEKING A CALMER AND MORE PEACEFUL LIFE."

The calmer, saner, more peaceful life I had longed to achieve for so long required that first I find the place of nothingness, the place of absolute peace in my own mind. I had found a machine that could help me get there. I was onto something big.

THE CAREER

What started as a hobby for me, a way to relax and ease my anxiety, has transformed my life in so many ways. I have been able to reduce my medication to taking it only as needed. At one time I was taking multiple prescription medications just to function, and I had to take an acid reducer to keep my heart burn down (a side effect of my medications). I no longer need to see a therapist weekly to work on my anxiety. In fact, I rarely get anxiety anymore, and when I do I know exactly what to do to relieve it. I see my counselor once a month now, but I use those sessions more for coaching than anything else. We work on a better future and creating a great plan rather than focusing on fixing issues.

Am I saying that if you float all will be cured for you? No, there isn't a cure-all for anything in life, and I urge you to seek out help and relief anywhere you can get it.

Every person is different, every situation is special, and the many things I've had to do to find peace were all worthwhile.

What I am saying is floating was the cure for what ailed me. It was the cure for my spinning thoughts, anxiety, hopelessness, and depression. It remains a cure for those issues. As long as I'm floating regularly, my life is stable, my mind is healthy, and my future is bright.

I truly believe that floating should be a staple for anyone seeking a calmer and more peaceful life. I cannot promise that you will see the results I did. But I can assure you that others have, and you'll hear from several of them in this book. The benefits of floating are vast. In my opinion, floating is the next wave of well-being for society at large. As we head further into a time of over-connectedness and over-stimulation, the float tank is the anecdote to that intake overload.

The day I built that first float tank in my basement, my life changed. First, through improved health and well-being, and then through a new dream. I wanted to bring this same peace of mind, this same in-house availability to other people. I wanted to share my new freedom.

Working with a couple of partners, I drew up the plans for a floatation tank that is portable and affordable for people to use in their homes. At the time, the idea of floating was becoming more mainstream, and float spas were opening in a few major cities.

Our newly formed company rode the wave of this new interest, and soon, I had made a career out of my hobby. We've made it possible for hundreds of people to float at home anywhere in the world, and I couldn't be happier. We make float tanks for the enthusiast who wants to float more than a few times a month at a float center, the people who want to float in the privacy of their home whenever they want. These people are improving themselves and in turn the world they live in. That's why we do it.

It's my life and my mission to bring the peace and freedom of floating to as many people as I can and to help the world discover the float cure.

Despite how important floating is in my life, I run into people all the time who still haven't heard of it. Or if they have, they shake their heads or roll their eyes and dismiss it as weird. "You don't *do* anything in there," people say.

I wrote this book to help you understand what floating is, what it can do for you, and how other people just like you are seeing their lives transformed for the better.

And I wrote this book to share my own story. Because floating is my cure, and it just might be yours too.

THE NOBLEST
PLEASURE IS
THE JOY OF
UNDERSTANDING.
-LEONARDO DA VINCI

CHAPTER 1
WHAT IS FLOATING?

The basic idea of floating is simple. First, you minimize or completely remove the sensory input to your brain. You just shut everything off—every signal to your brain from the outside world. The goal is to create an environment that allows for greater focus, deeper meditation, and more effective thought. It's hard to get really quiet and really still when your foot itches or your dog barks.

The first time I had a panic attack, I was in a Las Vegas hotel room. And I created this state of calm for a few minutes in the hotel bathtub. I had no idea that floating was a method for achieving a state of calm, much less for reducing stress and improving overall physical, mental, and emotional health.[1] All I knew was that I felt like I was losing my mind and the only thing I could think to do was climb into the bathtub to try and calm down.

With the warm water up over my ears, I found a

little peace in the midst of the chaos in my mind. The problem was that I couldn't keep the world out even in the bathtub. My phone rang, the water cooled, and I got goose bumps. The bathtub was a temporary fix. What I needed was a cure.

If I was going to truly quiet my mind, I needed total isolation.

"90%OFTHECENTRALNERVOUSSYSTEM'S WORKLOADISRELATEDTOGRAVITY,LIGHT, SOUND, AND TOUCH."

Most everyone has five senses: touch, sight, sound, taste, and smell. Taste and smell are easy to remove. You just go into a clean, empty room and don't eat anything, and they're gone. The real distractions come from touch, sight, and sound. These are the hardest to minimize and the ones floating aims to eliminate. If you're living a normal life, you're in a constant state of hearing, seeing, and feeling. It's just the way life is. It's how we function as human beings. Even if you're doing nothing but standing or sitting still, you are balancing your body, monitoring room noise, and processing your visual surroundings. Your brain is always scanning, computing, categorizing, and working away as it monitors your surroundings and your state of being. Well-trained monks have the power of a full-focus, zero-distraction mental state. The rest of us usually don't.

That is, unless we're floating.

THE FIRST FLOATERS

Floating was created by a man named John C. Lilly in 1954. Lilly was studying neurophysiology with the National Institute of Mental Health in Bethesda, Maryland. Basically, he conducted consciousness research. He looked for ways to alter reality, to dive deeper into the mind. His experiments involved isolating the brain from external stimuli. He determined that 90 percent of the central nervous system's workload is related to gravity, light, sound, and touch.

That means that 90 percent of the workload for your nervous system, including your brain, comes from your surroundings. So if you're awake, your nervous system is on high alert.

Lilly created the first float tank. Essentially, it was a pool of water that allowed a person to float upright. An underwater device covered the subject's head and supplied oxygen. Looking back now, I think it must have been a difficult way to achieve the effects of isolation compared to the current reclining float tanks, but it was a great start.

Lilly and his colleagues quickly became the first subjects of their own research, using the isolation tank and recording their experiences. In *Deep Self: Profound Relaxation and the Tank Isolation Technique* (1977), Lilly wrote: "All the average person has to do is to get into the tank in the darkness and silence and float around until he realizes he is programming everything that is happening inside his head. You are free of the physical world at that point and anything can happen inside your head because everything is governed by the laws of thought rather than the laws of the external world. So you can go to the limits of your conceptions."

This experimentation with consciousness and thought was intriguing to many during the '70s—mainly students. In the early days, Lilly would conduct workshops and allow students to try out the float tank. One of the young people at a Lilly lecture was Glenn Perry, a computer programmer at the time. Glenn was, by his own account, painfully shy. But after he stepped out of the isolation tank and Lilly asked him to share his experience, Glenn immediately began to speak in front of a large group of fellow attendees.

"I thought if something could make me that comfortable talking to people, it must be pretty incredible," Glenn told me. "When I came out of the tank the first time, the universe was a shimmering, vibrating energy system. My hearing was heightened, everything was sparkling. It's like I was in an altered state."

Glenn wanted to float again, as well as share his discovery with his friends, so he went home and figured out plans to build his own tank. "I would float before work each day," he says. "I'd go to work and on the freeway I would be in the slow lane wondering why everyone was going so fast. Whereas previously I was in the fast lane wondering why everyone was going so slow.

"For me, it has never been about what happens in the tank. It's always been about how I feel afterwards," Glenn says.

He began talking more about his transformation, and many people seemed interested. That's when it hit him: "I might as well make them for others. It shouldn't be much harder," he says. "I was so naïve."

A few years later, Lee Leibner, who was a teacher at the time, was a test subject in an isolation tank study. The tank she floated in was one that Glenn had built. They met at a party a couple days later and have been together for the forty years since. Lee even joined Glenn in his work with Lilly.

Today, the Perrys' company Samadhi is the longest running floating business in the world.

Of course, there were obstacles to the success of early floating. Amnesty International came down on people doing research on sensory deprivation, confusing the technique with torture. In the '80s, AIDS arrived, along with early misinformation and prejudice that frightened people away from shared tanks. And then there were all the weird looks and questions.

"When we first started telling people what we did," Glenn says, "they'd say, 'What? Why? What for?'"

The earliest adopters had to develop a language to use when talking about sensory deprivation, especially when the concept of deprivation took on a justifiably negative connotation to the public.

Fortunately, Lilly's team was working to make the experience easy and was experimenting with ocean water for better flotation. Glenn decided to add additional salt to the water, and eventually upped the percentage until he reached total saturation. The effect was huge! This heavily salted water increased a person's buoyancy and finally allowed for an effortless reclining float.

This also allowed the group of pioneering colleagues to start referring to the practice as floating.

"One of the things that was so attractive to people, especially those who couldn't float [in fresh water]," Lee says, "was that first sensation when you get in and you lie down and you get pushed up to the surface. People were very attracted to that sensation of floating, of being held by the water. So we started to use the word floating."

Later, a researcher named Dr. Rod Borrie coined the term REST, which stood for Restricted Environmental Stimulation Therapy or Technique.

MY QUEST FOR A TANK

The day I stumbled upon a video of Joe Rogan talking about floating, he used words like isolation and deprivation, which sounded scary. But it also began to sound irresistible.

As I watched the video, I listened to the then host of *Fear Factor* talk about the adventure into his own mind that he took every time he floated. Riddled with anxiety, panic, and depression, I wanted so desperately to go on that adventure in my own mind. I could envision myself launching into mental space and leaving the world behind. It was romantic and thrilling.

I watched the video every night before bed— sometimes twice. I would go to sleep with it playing in my mind and wake up only to hit play again. I don't know why I obsessed over it like I did, but I knew floating was my answer. The powerful mind that had taken me into an extreme hell was now going to take me on a journey through space and ecstasy. I was going to unleash my brain in a positive way.

Well, the dream proved to be much harder than I had planned. I researched float centers online, and I found that the closest one to Salt Lake City where I lived was in Las Vegas. There were very few float centers back in 2011, and they were only located in major cities. I remember budgeting a trip to go floating and thinking *If I end up liking it, I won't have the money left over to buy a tank.* Then I thought, *I know I'll like it. What's not to like?*

I decided to jump straight to tank ownership. I had no idea, to quote Glenn Perry, how naïve I really was.

In 2011 buying an affordable float tank for your home was like buying an affordable airplane. Basically the good new ones weren't affordable, and the stuff that was affordable was, well, kind of scary looking. I remember shopping online and seeing only two tanks priced under $10,000. One was a custom built tank that had been pulled apart. It was covered in salt and looked like it had survived since the '70's. The next one was this big plastic pill looking thing that reminded me of a bread loaf with army tank-style access. There was no way it would fit through my door. I chose the one I could pull apart and got a quote to ship it. The tank itself was $6,000. Add in $2,000 for shipping, and I would have to spend a whopping $8,000. If I was going to afford something like that, I knew I'd better start saving.

Sometime during my shopping period I remember thinking "It's just a pitch black tub with a cover." Surely I could build something like that. I had grown up building skate ramps and helping out my dad and grandpa building stuff around the house. You could say I was handy.

I ordered a farming fertilizer tank—at 4-foot by 8-foot it was just the right size—and paid only $500. While I waited for it to arrive, I spent long nights awake building my tank in my head. I would lie on my back in bed looking up into the darkness and thinking about how the thing was going to go together.

I thought of using aquarium parts to heat and clean the water. I planned to frame around the tank and insulate it just like a house. And since I'd have to saw the tank in half to fit it into my basement, I came up with a tanning bed design with a lifting top.

Finally, the tank arrived. I made a trip to Home Depot for supplies, and I set to work.

My roommate thought I was nuts. He and his girlfriend would come down to the basement to see if I was still alive. They politely asked what it was, and rather than try to make it sound normal, I said, "It's a weird meditation chamber. Don't worry about it."

Without going into all the details, let me just say that inventions always work better in my mind than they do in real life. I had to change the hinging, change the covering, change the heater, change the lighting, change just about everything! There were many Home Depot trips when I had to explain why I needed three heavy duty hinges that could support a 200-pound toy box lid, or why I needed 30 feet of garage seal to help close off my hot tub lid, or why I needed my fish to have 94 degree water.

Looking back, I probably would have been better off telling the truth. But at the time I figured explaining the truth would take too long.

After many long nights and confusing Home Depot trips, the idea was reality. I ordered 800 pounds of Epsom salt and added it to the shallow water. After a few days, the aquarium heater had warmed the salt water. I was ready to take it for a test drive.

WHATHAPPENSWHENYOUFLOAT

The experience and the effects vary according to your reasons for floating, but the method is essentially the same.

The tank is filled with ten inches of heavily salted water. The salt helps you to float easier, so even people who have trouble floating in a pool or in the ocean find it easy to float in a tank. The water is set at the exact temperature as your skin. What this means is that when you lie back and bob to the top of the water, you don't feel anything. It's like being suspended in mid-air with no gravity and no wind. To keep out sight and sound, the tank has a light-proof cover and most people wear ear plugs.

"ONCEYOULETGO,THEMAGICHAPPENS."

When I describe the experience to some people, they feel nervous. It's a normal reaction. But let me tell you, the first time people step into a tank and lie back and feel the full experience of nothing—no noise, no interruptions, no nagging smells or sounds to distract them—they usually are amazed at how much freedom and peace they feel.

I encourage everyone who hasn't floated to try floating at least three times. Here's why: On your first float you are likely going to be highly alert and a little concerned because you're in a foreign environment. Again, this is perfectly normal. Most people spend their first session getting comfortable with their surroundings. On your second float, you'll be familiar with the process and you'll likely have a relaxing time. By the time your third float comes around, you'll be comfortable, know what to expect, and really be able to relax and let go.

Once you let go, the magic happens. When you're not worried about sinking, falling asleep, or breathing, you really start to have insightful experiences.

Floating is a maintenance therapy.

Yes, the experience of floating is helpful—even once. But for me and many others it's become an ongoing part of our overall health and wellness plan, much like exercise.

I prefer now to float weekly, while others float multiple times a week or twice a month. The frequency is up to you and should be adjusted according to your needs.

For example, if you float for pain relief, you'll benefit

from being in a tank multiple times a week. You can compare the relief and satisfaction you'll get to that you receive from a chiropractor appointment or massage.

People like me float for focus and calmness, and we get a similar feeling as that from a massage or yoga session. I feel balanced, relaxed, and rejuvenated.

"ITWASLIKEAPURESHOTOFMEDITATION AND MIND EXPLORATION."

Some people float to think more clearly and enhance learning or creativity. They compare the mental clarity after floating to the stimulation and insight they feel after meeting with a mentor or a study group.

Athletes float to visualize and prepare for their next competition and to help their bodies recover more quickly from intense training. These people often compare the feeling after a float to a smooth practice session and a sense of preparedness.

Whatever your reasons, you likely will find positive benefits from floating. I'm always amazed at the experiences I hear, and I'm encouraged that while floating is the same for all of us, its unique effects seem tailored just for me.

MY FIRST REAL FLOAT

You know that little voice inside your head that directs you through your day? After a few minutes floating in my new tank, it was like I was hanging out with that voice. I was fully alone with myself. No sights, sounds, tastes, smells, or sensations whatsoever.

As I lay in that fertilizer tank, my heart raced. I remember lying there with my eyes open and thinking, "There's nothing to do!" It took a while to settle in, but I really enjoyed having my eyes wide open and thinking. I enjoyed the feeling of falling through space and not having any boundaries.

At first my brain was grasping for stimuli, but after a while it calmed down and settled into the experience. I got really calm and really peaceful. I would sometimes have an itch or an adjustment of my arms or legs, but otherwise it was like being with myself in a way I hadn't experienced before. I was with my true self. For me it was like a pure shot of meditation and mind exploration. I was in love with nothing!

I ended my first float feeling like there was so much more to experience, but I needed more time in the tank.

I wanted so much more, but it wasn't going to come in one float. I still compare it to the feeling of going to the gym. You always feel better after one trip, but when you make it a habit, you truly start to feel the results.

Floating often was no problem for me now that I had a float tank in my basement. I floated almost every day right when I would wake up and sometimes at the end of the day. I was noticeably changing. I remember a co-worker telling me I seemed different, like I was on something that made me extra calm. I was on something alright. I was on Float. And I was determined to spread the word.

As I built my tank, I had documented all of my plans, mistakes, and triumphs. I had the whole process on film in some form or another. So I put all of my plans online, along with pictures and video of my process. I quickly discovered that I wasn't the only weird one who was obsessed with floating.

People started popping up from all over the world wanting to float but without options that worked for them. The traffic on my website blew up, and I started receiving a ton of email. I improved the plans online and turned my one-time basement project into a thriving hobby.

Meeting and helping other people who were also seeking a solution in floating was so gratifying to me. I was able to put my own experience to use for others and found a supportive, adventurous community in the process. I helped people set up float tanks in their homes and in newly formed float centers. In fact, there are floating professionals today who have a tank just like the one in my basement in their float center thanks to those online plans.

This process of helping people build tanks is how I met William Hill, my future partner at Zen Float Co. William reached out to me with questions on floating and tank building design. We became friends, and eventually he felt close enough to me to share his revolutionary idea: building a float tank from waterproof canvas.

William's idea absolutely blew my mind. I had looked at all the typical methods of building float tanks and had built the most affordable one to date. Then someone came in and exploded my ideas into oblivion.

Canvas was the answer. I just knew it, and William

did, too. We quickly began work on what is known today as the Float Tent. It took us a couple years, but we finally created a good working prototype and were able to keep the price under $2,000.

We had a feeling that this was going to change floating forever.

THE FLOAT BOOM

I was sitting at The Float Conference in 2013 looking around at the hundreds of people in the room. Ashkahn Jahromi and Graham Talley from FloatOn in Portland put on an incredible conference every year. It's an awesome event, jam-packed with float shop owners, researchers, and enthusiasts.

That day, Ashkahn was asking the crowd to raise their hands to show when they first heard of floating. He started with 1970, and a handful of people raised their hands. I think mainly the REST researchers and of course Glenn and Lee Perry who worked with John C. Lilly.

Then Ashkahn asked who had first heard of floating in the '80's, and another few people raised their hands. Then '90's, 2000, 2010—still only a small fraction were holding up their hands.

I remember thinking, *What's the deal? How on earth could it be this new to so many people when such a huge crowd was enthusiastic enough to fly around the world to be here*

Ashkahn said 2011, and a third of the room raised their hands. He said 2012 and another third, then 2013 and the final third raised their hands. This to me was truly incredible and a clear signal that the world is changing.

Today, floating as a practice is exploding. In the summer of 2011, there wasn't a single float center in the entire state of Utah. Now there are three just within a short drive from my house. I used to mention floating to people, knowing that they'd have no clue what I was talking about. Now, I know there's a pretty good chance they've heard of it. Ten years ago, you wouldn't have turned up many search results online using the keywords "float tank." Today, there are thousands of float sites. The industry is exploding.

People everywhere, in almost every country, are floating now. If you live in even a small- to mid-sized city, you likely have a float center. Education and enthusiasm are rapidly expanding. No doubt we will see better funded studies come out with more clout in the health industry. We will likely see health insurance start to cover floating if it hasn't already. The future is so bright, and I'm so thankful to be a part of it.

One day people will look back at the weird folks who were trying to spread the weird hobby and think "that's pretty awesome." And that makes me proud.

A SHIFT IN SOCIETY

I believe a large contributor to the new popularity of floating is our society's growing interest in natural and holistic health approaches. There has been a dramatic shift in the number of people who are looking for these so-called alternative therapies and remedies over the past several years. What prompted this shift?

Many in my generation have seen how Western medicine and health practices alone aren't enough to treat every situation and every person. We grew up feeling like there must be more to our health than a scan or a chart full of data. While our parents' generation often took a doctor's advice as the only option, we began to suspect that there should be more to it. After all, we saw truly unwell people who looked perfectly healthy, according to the numbers.

"(FLOATING)WASIMPROVINGMYOVERALL WELL-BEING IN WAYS I HAD NEVER IMAGINED."

We've searched for the answers within. We've opened ourselves to other teachings, other traditions, and other ideas for how to be fully healthy—mind, body, and spirit.

This trend runs along a pendulum track that I think most human nature follows. We are always in pursuit of what we don't have, so we tend to swing back and forth between options. You can see this movement in food production clearly.

At one time food was much harder to come by and much harder to store. People would die of starvation because food would rot and become scarce. When we developed processed foods in the early 1900's, things really started to change. Now we could create a food that would stay good for months and even years, often without refrigeration. These innovations solved many problems, but not all of them.

The processed food offered high amounts of short-term energy. Soon the high sugar content in heavily processed foods eaten on a regular basis started to affect people's body weights. You could get a day's worth of calories in one meal. The food that stayed edible for months also became hard for our bodies to process. The high amounts of sugar cranked up our fat storage. Without proper digestion and the continued addition of processed foods, we gained more and more weight as a society.

Many in our generation and those after it are keenly aware that while food technology is helpful in many cases, it needs to be balanced with other less processed approaches. Recognizing the problems caused by dependence on processed foods—obesity, diabetes, heart disease—many people are leading the charge toward whole and natural foods that our bodies are adapted to eating and are able to digest well. The pendulum has swung too far, and we're trying hard these days to swing it back.

A similar story can be told about medicine, which used to consist of plants, herbs, and extracts. Science and modern medicine are invaluable, and I'm in no way advocating that we abandon the scientific innovations that serve us individually and as a society. Steve Jobs battled pancreatic cancer through purely alternative means, despite the fact that he knew we had proven medical treatments available to fight and reduce his type of cancer. He later realized he had made a mistake, but it was too late.

However, relying entirely on modern medicine may not be the answer either. When doctors are performing surgery to remove fat that was gained through an addiction to food, there's a serious underlying spiritual and psychological problem that isn't being treated. In fact, it's potentially being aggravated.

I truly believe that our job as healthy, whole individuals is to sort through the options and try to achieve balance. We must ask ourselves what works, what the side effects are, as well as what are the odds and the outcomes.

As I adopted floating into my life more and more until I had developed a habit, I came to realize that it was improving my overall well-being in ways I had never imagined. As you read through the rest of this book, I hope you'll note what outcomes might be possible for you as well. Not only so you'll be encouraged to try floating or increase your involvement in this incredible practice, but also to make informed choices about your health.

TENSION IS WHO
YOU THINK YOU
SHOULD BE.
RELAXATION IS
WHO YOU ARE.
-CHINESE PROVERB

CHAPTER 2
REDUCE STRESS

Many people ask me what "the point" is of floating. They understand that it sounds relaxing, but so does sitting on the sofa watching their favorite TV show.

The benefits of floating are absolutely life-altering. Especially when it comes to stress.

Unlike many other forms of relaxation or escape, floating not only aids relaxation, it also changes the way you look at life. It takes you from a place of outward focus to a place of inward focus. That's a rare thing in this world.

Our society wires us from a young age to look outward for happiness. From the time we're about 2 years old, we focus on *having*. Whether it's a toy, treat, or game, we learn that getting things equals happiness. There's nothing wrong with getting things and being happy about it, but most of us know deep down that's only a part of happiness. There's a bigger part that is based on inner contentment, on a peace that can only be achieved through introspection and understanding.

If you're like most people, your life is filled with distractions, demands, and endless stresses that seem to run your life. Whether it comes from outside of you or it begins in your own mind with self-defeating thoughts or even conditions like ADHD, the negative impact of stress can derail your goals and ruin your health.

In my own life, stress led me to seek temporary solutions and quick-fixes. I found myself growing more and more frightened, on edge, and withdrawn. Rather than address the source of the stress or find a healthy way to achieve inner calm in the midst of it, I used alcohol, caffeine, and denial to keep myself going.

What I discovered the hard way is stress doesn't go away if you just ignore it. The circumstance you're worried about might resolve, but the negative effects of that stress on your mind and body will remain unless you make some changes.

Think of it like hitting the reset button. You've got to clear out all the junk that you accumulate along the way or else it builds up until you reach a breaking point.

To hit my own reset button, I started meditating. The sense of quiet, calm, and self-acceptance I found were liberating. But I could only get so far with meditation practice. I had trouble quieting my mind consistently and needed help achieving the level of peace that was truly healing for me.

That's where floating came in.

But before we get further into the effects of floating

on stress, let's take a look at where your stress is coming from. Because if you can reduce it, your floating routine—and any other methods of stress-reduction you may use—will be much more effective.

IDENTIFY YOUR STRESS

Stress is a crucial part of growing and achieving as a person. We don't want to eliminate all forms of stress. Instead, our goal is to minimize the forms of stress that pose hazards to our overall well-being.

In the '50's, a physiologist named Hans Selye identified our basic reactions to what he termed "stressors." His early findings led future researchers to categorize stress into two main types: eustress and distress.[2]

Eustress is considered positive. This is the type of stress that causes you to work harder, strive longer, and feel motivated to succeed. It's usually short-term, and in healthy individuals, it's manageable.[3] It makes us uncomfortable enough to get something done, but isn't outside of our coping ability. This type of good stress is usually exciting and will improve our performance. Think buying a home, getting married, moving, or starting a new career.

Demands like these, which we put on ourselves, cause a good kind of stress. We have the ability to channel that stress into action and achieve what we set out to do. Take, for example, the goal of losing weight. There is a certain amount of stress in the fact that you feel out of shape. That feeling of stress motivates you to get yourself to the gym or choose the healthy food option for lunch. If you never cared or never felt stress over the weight gain, you might never have the inner drive you need to make a change. So stress isn't always bad.

Distress, on the other hand, is caused by something that feels overwhelming or unpleasant and is outside of your ability to cope. It leads to worry, anxiety, poor performance, and other physical and mental problems.[4]

Common sources of distress are losing a loved one, career setbacks, legal problems, illness or injury, and relationship difficulties. But the source may also be something less noticeable, such as a long-term fear or conflict that you think you're managing but is slowly building to derail you.

Fears are considered internal stressors, and they can get quite toxic if they're not kept in check. Perhaps you have anxiety in social situations (social anxiety), fear of public speaking as you prepare for a presentation, fear of flying or heights, or just a general fear and unease about the future. Everyone has fears, and they flash across our conscious mind from time to time. It's the healthy way we stay aware of threats and challenges in our lives.

But these same fears can become negative once we start to make them habitual. So ask yourself: Are you worrying about a particular event that's coming up, or do you worry constantly no matter what events are coming up? Do you have a phobia that is limiting your behavior and making it hard to do certain things you enjoy, connect with others, or build your career? This negative kind of stress can steal your peace of mind and rob you of a bright future if left unchecked.

"IT'S UP TO YOU TO MANAGE YOUR STRESS AND MAINTAIN YOUR WELL-BEING NO MATTER WHAT'S GOING ON IN YOUR LIFE."

The negative impact of stress has been shown to worsen and up your risk of high blood pressure, heart disease, depression, obesity, diabetes, asthma, Alzheimer's disease, and gastrointestinal problems.[5] Much of this is believed to be due to increased cortisol levels produced by high levels of stress.

For an issue that so severely threatens our health, we often pay very little attention to it until we are forced to change.

Distress has a tendency to show up in negative emotions. Here are some signs you're overloaded with distress:

- You feel nervous over small situations.
- Little things cause unreasonable amounts of anger.
- You feel anxious or depressed for no apparent reason.
- You are unable to concentrate.

Distress is usually the cause of people's mental and physical problems, but even too much of a good thing can turn bad. Eustress, while usually motivating and positive, can come too often or too intensely for a person to handle.

What if you got married, moved to a new city, and started a new job all in one month? All of these life changes are positive and would normally drive you to become your best, but in a compact amount of time, they become overwhelming and detrimental.

My grandfather told me a story about his time in the U.S. Army during basic training. Basic training usually lasts for ten weeks. They put the new soldiers under just the right amount of mental and physical stress to help them grow the most they can in the shortest amount of time possible.

Well, when my grandfather went to basic training, the Army was preparing for war. They didn't have a full ten weeks to put the new recruits through standard training, so they packed ten weeks into eight. It ended up having the opposite effect from what they hoped. Too much positive stress too fast wore the soldiers down. By the end of the eight weeks, the soldiers were actually doing fewer pushups and sit-ups, and they were running slower than they had in the first week. They were overloaded, and what should have been positive stress turned negative.

Whether it's eustress or distress, internal or external, the pressures of life can distract you from what's important in your day and hijack your attention and your health. It's up to you to manage your stress and maintain your well-being no matter what's going on in your life.

So let's take a closer look at what types of external and internal stressors cause the most damage on a regular basis and talk about some ways you can manage it.

INTAKE OVERLOAD

Today's world offers countless conveniences, but sometimes all they seem to do is create more distractions, more stress, and less time for what really matters. We are over-connected and overloaded. With one click I can find out what my best friend from third grade had for lunch or how my mom's cousin is treating her daughter's bee sting.

The opportunity to connect with loved ones is wonderful, but the distraction that too much information causes in our lives is beyond ridiculous.

"INTAKEOVERLOADISINESCAPABLEUNLESS YOUHAVETHECONFIDENCETOSTEPAWAY FROMYOURDEVICESANDDISAPPOINTAFEW PEOPLE."

Eric Schmidt, CEO of Google, told crowds at the 2010 Techonomy Conference that we create as much information in two days as we did from the dawn of man through 2003. And that rate is only accelerating.

Not too many years ago, you might meet at most two or three distractions at your desk: someone knocking on your door or the landline ringing. If you just took your phone off the hook and put a Do Not Disturb sign on your door, you could have uninterrupted time for focus and purposeful action.

Now, your phone probably has your work, social, and family lives all coming at you at once through different forms of communication like email, texts, tweets, posts, and phone calls. We have to actually work at overcoming these external distractions to our real work.

Every day, I spend time working to intentionally shut off what I call intake overload.

Today, everyone you know—and most of the people you have ever known—have access to you in some way, no matter where you are. Do you realize how many potential distractions and stresses that can create?

There's a high cost for allowing others to hijack your schedule. Whether it's someone's quick question, a drift into online land, or the buzz of your phone, interruptions cost you time and attention. Think about it: Every time you stop to check the latest notification, how long does it take you to get back into the focused zone you just abandoned? Do you find yourself getting up for a snack, deciding to check email, or starting an entirely new task?

After you get back from your break or work your way back into the zone, tally how much time you're actually spending on that interruption—is it five, ten, fifteen minutes? Just to check your phone. Or answer a question that could have waited until the next meeting.

Regardless of what you do for a living, you are a firefighter, and everyone expects you to be available 24 hours a day.

Intake overload is inescapable unless you have the confidence to step away from your devices and disappoint a few people.

Look, I decided a long time ago to stop being so available all the time. I used to keep my phone on a 24-hour "do not disturb" so that the only thing that distracted me was my choice to look at it. Of course, some of that is changing now that I'm a father, but everyone has to set their own boundary with this practice.

Your smartphone should have a feature that allows

you to either put your phone in a do not disturb mode (iPhone) or blocking mode (Android) to reduce the number of interruptions you receive via phone and text messaging. You can also select to turn off notifications from apps.

Again, some of these options won't work for every person, but I highly recommend that you at least take advantage of this option for social networks. Do you really need to know right away if someone "likes" the picture of your dog? You can still find out this information, but if you turn off notifications, you'll be checking your networks on your own time table and not someone else's. Give some thought to the kind of interruptions that are worth spending valuable time on every day.

Once you implement these changes, you'll have to train others to respect your new communication boundaries. If you've been the one who's always available, you're performing the role of a firefighter or at least the 911 operator. You're on call 24/7. And unless you're a medical professional or an actual firefighter, you are not required to be available at a moment's notice. Our society trains us to be this way. Because of this pervasive habit, most of us feel guilty when we don't respond immediately to a message or answer a phone call. I used to feel like I was constantly letting people down by not being available as soon as they emailed.

After I decided to set my own boundaries and take back control of my schedule, I had to take time to train people on what to expect. This meant first helping them understand I was going to be available only during certain times. You can choose to write this information in your email or make a call to the important people in your life to let them know you're making some changes in your communication habits. I now respond within 48 hours, and I've found that everyone who adjusted to this change with me is positively impacted by it as well.

External demands and distractions are only as stressful as you allow them to be. Take control of your schedule and your time, and you will probably find—as I have—that some of your peace of mind naturally returns.

ADHD FOR EVERYONE

A common source of internal stress is Attention-Deficit/Hyperactivity Disorder (ADHD). Recent surveys by the Centers for Disease Control and Prevention show that, 11 percent of children 4 to 17 years old were diagnosed with ADHD in 2011, up from 7.8 percent in 2003.[6] Many of these children will carry the disorder into adulthood.

Essentially, ADHD is a problem of being unable to focus, being overactive, being unable to control impulses, or a combination of these symptoms.

What I find remarkable is this is exactly the description of the habits we are creating with our technology. We are training people to have disordered thinking.

Ask yourself honestly: If you hear your phone buzz, how long can you go without checking it?

I'm going to bet most people would come in at five minutes tops. You might feel like you can control your behavior, but I'm going to bet your habits say otherwise.

Just because we can do all of these things at the touch of a button and within the space of a couple minutes doesn't mean we should. We've got to learn to treat our time and concentration as valuable.

Floating is an ideal solution. It helps you stay focused, on task and present, no matter what. And for people who deal with the very real symptoms of ADHD on a regular basis, a floating routine might have similar effects.

Spencer Fossier, owner of NOLA Float Tanks, first floated in 2014. Since then, he's not only adopted a regular float schedule to deal with symptoms of ADHD and back pain but has also opened his own float center.

Diagnosed and medicated for ADHD in the fourth grade, Spencer spent years feeling hopeless and misunderstood. Now he says, "It has opened me up immensely." His symptoms are alleviated, and he chooses to stay off medication.

But Spencer says floating also helped him come to peace with his diagnosis and the struggles he went through as a child. "Whereas before, I kind of was this angry little kid, was just frustrated that no one else got it and I was just a victim of situations. More than anything else, floating has helped me realize I'm just responsible for my own life and decisions. And not only that, but I'm not responsible for the way that other people react to me."

He says that regardless of why you're doing it, you

should keep an open mind and that every float is different, even for him. "Everyone needs to do it," he says. "It's a life-changing experience. You will learn more about yourself in those forty-five minutes to an hour than most people have ever sat down to think about in their entire lives."

Whether you suffer from ADHD or simply the disordered thinking of an overloaded society, floating can help you move to a more peaceful place.

BEING YOUR OWN WORST ENEMY

I know a lot of people who are overscheduled, but I was not one of them. I had the opposite problem: lack of planning.

I would have tons to do with no plan or division of time in which to do them. I would work, work, work, but I never organized my day to include self-care. Instead, I would take on unlimited projects, assignments, and family obligations because nothing else was planned. By the end of the week, I realized I didn't have any down time for myself. I ended up burned out and out of time.

Many people underestimate just how valuable relaxation is to their well-being. In many ways, our society has tabooed relaxation. Most Americans have a certain degree of guilt when it comes to doing nothing.

We know days of doing nothing feel great. We know a weekend with no plans revives us. And we know a vacation can make us feel alive and happy in the face of high levels of stress. Yet nobody seems to make relaxation a priority.

I think that to really put relaxation as a priority in your life, you need to first pay attention and realize just how valuable it is. Next time you relax, watch what it does to you and make a mental note. The next time you have a relaxing weekend, journal about it. The next time you're flying home from a trip, spend the flight contemplating how you feel and why.

Then put those observations into action and make a point to schedule relaxation into your day, your week, and your month. Rather than allowing yourself to run from one thing to the next, always saying yes and never determining what's really best for you, intentionally schedule down time.

Arrange your task list in such a way that allows for activities to be swapped out, depending on how you're feeling. For example, I'm writing this book, so I block out sections of time during each week to write. If I happen to start feeling burned out during the week, I can skip or reduce one of these writing sessions in exchange for something to help myself unwind. These types of flexible tasks are crucial to maintaining your mental health and your productivity.

If everything on your calendar is mandatory or requires you to meet an obligation to other people, you might be setting yourself up for burnout. But if you leave slack in your schedule on things that are moveable, you'll be able to manage your stress as you go.

Another issue that causes stress is self-doubt. We all have fears and negative tapes that play in our minds. One of the biggest is self-doubt based on what other people think of us.

"OFTEN, YOURSELF-DOUBTISINSPIREDBY AFEAROFWHATOTHERSTHINKOFYOU."

As you begin to make changes in how you protect your time and build relaxation into your routine, you will probably encounter a big flare up of this issue. I've witnessed the guilt that people go through when they take a day off, need to leave work for something relaxing like a massage or a float session, or decide not to return a phone call right away. When you boil that concern down, it really comes to wanting to be liked, which is a stress management issue.

Wanting to be liked has got to be one of the most crippling and toxic desires we have as human beings. At one time it was essential to fit in, to be part of the tribe for survival. Now this desire causes us to overwork, overcommit, and do things we don't want to do all in the name of being liked and accepted by others.

If you know what to do to take care of yourself and you fail to do it because of others, you've got a big problem. Often, your self-doubt is inspired by a fear of what others think of you. Here's how I've reframed this issue for myself. It may help you too.

In his book *The Slight Edge: The Secret to a Successful Life*, Jeff Olson describes reading a magazine article that disturbed him. The article reported that at the average funeral, only about ten people cry. Olson writes: "That's it? You mean I go through my entire life, spend years going through all these trials and tribulations and achievements and joys and heartbreaks—and at the end of it, there are only ten people who care enough to cry?"

To put this in perspective, you might be living your life with more stress and worry to please people who may not even show up to your funeral, let alone cry! For me, hearing this changed everything. I no longer worry about what others think of me, outside of those I know will be crying such as my closest family and friends. The rest of the world can just deal with the fact that they're not happy with me because of some commitment I didn't take or a long weekend I took for myself.

You are ultimately responsible for your own happiness and well-being. Isn't it time you stopped worrying so much about what other people think and take control of it?

FIGHT STRESS FROM THE INSIDE OUT

The biggest key to reducing my stress level has been to start from the inside out, building strength and peace of mind that I can then take into the world. Essentially I fight intake overload, self-doubt, and anxiety through a series of calculated actions—the most important of which is floating—that are all intended to create calm and stability inside my mind and body. With this kind of foundation, both external and internal sources of stress are much easier to withstand and much less damaging.

Floating is the opposite of intake overload.

In fact, it's almost the total elimination of intake.

Let's think again about how we take in sensory information: sight, hearing, smell, touch, and taste. No matter what you're doing in life, even sleeping, your senses are being affected. Even in the most comfortable bed with the perfect comforter, your body is fighting the pull of gravity, your skin is warm or cold, you brush against fabric, and you probably hear some house noise. The point I'm making is even in a very relaxed and comfortable state, your mind and body are processing information about your surroundings.

Floating was created with the hopes of eliminating all that input, and it has come close. Floating has reduced sensory input more than any other environment in the history of mankind. Sight has been eliminated with the use of a pitch black tank. Gravity has been nearly eliminated with the high concentration of salt water that allows your body to float on the water's surface. Smell has been eliminated because of the controlled closed tank. Sound has been reduced so much that with earplugs you can barely hear your heartbeat.

In a world where we are overrun with sources of intake that stress our minds and bodies, floating is the technology that will balance our state of overload.

This is especially true for individuals who find that they are more sensitive to input than others. For example, I've always felt sensitive to change and usually feel things before other people I know. It's my sensitive nature that has caused me so much anxiety and panic. But it has also allowed me insight into what is coming so I can make better decisions. Sensitivity isn't good or bad, it just is.

However, for people who are sensitive like me, intake overload can be a source of great discomfort and anxiety. Fortunately, I found floating, and it has helped me strengthen my reserves. Because beyond the healing calm I experience when I float, as Spencer touched on previously, there is a general adjustment in my attitude and approach to life.

"FLOATINGPRODUCESANEFFECTSIMILAR TO MEDITATION."

Other people experience this shift as well. It's as if upon entering the float tank, you open yourself to a more peaceful state of mind and that leads to a more peaceful state of being when you're done. Your reactions are tempered, your feelings are more balanced, and your life tends to calm down.

I love what Dr. Rod Borrie says: "When you cut out external stimulus, it's a refocusing."

Rod has spent the last forty years in the field of psychological research and practice. He has worked with sensory deprivation since coining the term REST (Restricted Environmental Stimulation Therapy) with Peter Suedfeld in the '70s. He's the former President of IRIS (the International REST Investigators Society), and is one of the only people actively conducting float tank research today through his Fibromyalgia Flotation Project.

Rod compares floating to biofeedback but without the machinery. The goal of biofeedback is to use electronic monitoring to train someone to acquire voluntary control of what is usually an automatic bodily function, such as breathing or a pain response. Many people get the same results through a floating practice.

Often when someone floats for the first time, they have a kind of awakening to their state of mind. When all sensory input stops and nervousness dissipates, the body relaxes. Rod explains: "It says, 'Hey, there's nothing happening here. I'm safe.' And the body self-regulates. That state is one of deep relaxation." He says that when someone experiences that for the first time, they commonly emerge from the tank and say, "Wow, I didn't realize I was so stressed."

This kind of awakening to your body and mind is powerful, and many people describe a resulting shift in perspective that is profoundly satisfying.

FLOATING FOR MEDITATION

As I've said before, you can have many different experiences in a float tank, from meditation to relaxation, from a think tank session to a relief and recovery session. The possibilities are up to you, and you decide what you're after. But it's clear that the meditative aspect of floating is most beneficial to stress relief.

For me, the relief first came in the form of guided meditation outside the tank. And I'm not alone. The number of people who have adopted meditation as a stress reduction technique is growing. The latest data from the National Health Interview Survey in 2012, reports that about 18 million U.S. adults practice meditation. That's

8 percent of the population.[7]

Floating produces an effect similar to meditation. "Something about the floating stops the racing mind," Rod says. "It stops the obsessing about worry. Because when you come out of the tank, the closest mental state that I can find to it is mindfulness meditation."

Graham Talley, co-founder and CEO of Portland-based Float On, agrees. "You pretty much put yourself into a hypnogogic state. Self-hypnosis is incredibly easy in the float tank." Graham, who is the co-founder of Float Conference and the Float Center Workshop, says that floating neutralizes both the external and internal factors that cause stress. "The float tank is cutting out both sides of that equation and letting you remember what it was like to be a normal version of yourself. Just a human without the outside world and all those things that were stressing you out."

Some of the earliest REST researchers discovered that floating creates reliable changes in our psychological and physiological states, including an improved ability to manage stress.[8]

Remember the elevated cortisol levels associated with increased stress that can cause problems with in all areas of the body? Floating results in proven reduction of cortisol levels even in comparison to other relaxation techniques, such as sitting quietly in a dimly lit room.[9]

Additional studies have shown floating's beneficial impact on hypertension or high blood pressure, a common symptom of stress. In fact, the patients' blood pressure not only dropped immediately after each float session, but remained lower for up to nine months.[10]

ENHANCING MEDITATION DURING A FLOAT

For some people, the first few times in a float tank might not be as relaxing as for others. This could be a result of fear or discomfort with the process, and it's completely normal. While I loved the experience from the beginning, I too have struggled sometimes with getting my mind to shut off. So I've developed a few techniques to kick start my meditative state while in the tank. If you have fear about floating, these might help you relax and settle into the experience.

"FLOATING TAKES YOUR BRAIN OUT OF THE CHAOS SOCIETY HAS CREATED AND PLACES IT INTO ITS NATURAL STATE OF PEACE AND STRESS-FREE HARMONY."

Here are a few ideas you might try:

- *Concentrated visual focus:*

  In standard meditation, this practice involves focusing on an item like a candle flame or a sacred object. Of course, in a pitch black float tank, that's hard to do. But the truth is when you're in the tank, even in the dark, your eyes perceive things. Perhaps it's a small dot, circle, or flare in your blank vision. Try not to think about what these shapes look like but just watch them. This method helps me to calm my thoughts and focus on being present.

- *Concentrated aural focus:*

You can also use the concentrated focus method on a sound. If you have audio in your tank, you can throw on a track of a gong or nature sounds. You can even make the sound yourself. Try speaking the "ohm" sound in a slow rhythm. Focus on the sound, and it will help you enter a meditative state. The key is staying absolutely in the moment and bringing your mind back to the sound if it wanders—and it will. Don't get frustrated when this happens. Just take a breath and bring it back. This is supposed to be a peaceful practice, remember?

- *Chanting a mantra:*

A mantra can be one word or a phrase of your choosing. I use the "ohm" sound, but you can pick anything short, simple, and meaningful to you. Recite it over and over and over as you float. I've found this practice leads to a thoughtless, effortless state that is proven to offer many benefits.

- *Counting backwards:*

This simple technique is one of the first things I did in a float tank to help clear my mind of its chaos. I count backwards from one hundred to zero. If I lose track of my count, I start over. As I count, I watch my breath come in and out and time it with the counting. So I count ninety-nine, breath in and out, count ninety-eight then breathe in and out, count ninety-seven then breathe in and out. By the time I get to zero, which takes a while, my mind is in a different realm.

From your first few times in a float tank, you'll realize the possibilities of introspection and self-improvement the experience makes available to you. You'll see the benefit of finding peace and practicing peace. You'll discover that same peace leaves the tank with you and starts to affect how you perceive and interact with the world around you.

I believe your life is a reflection of your inner state, and without a doubt I believe that floating affects your inner state, permanently, in fact. Floating takes your brain out of the chaos society has created and places it into its natural state of peace and stress-free harmony.

OUT OF SUFFERING HAVE EMERGED THE STRONGEST SOULS; THE MOST MASSIVE CHARACTERS ARE SEARED WITH SCARS.

-KHALIL GIBRAN

CHAPTER 3
BUILD A SHIELD AGAINST ANXIETY AND DEPRESSION

Mental illness touches just about every family in the United States. It wreaks havoc on our relationships, destroys careers, and takes lives. While medical and pharmaceutical research has come a long way in developing treatments, there are many alternative treatments available that might offer more hope.

More than 18 percent of adults in this country suffer from some form of mental illness. Among the most common are anxiety disorders, depression, and post-traumatic stress disorder.[11]

After trying countless solutions for my own struggles, I finally found permanent relief in floating.

My mental health is one of the primary reasons I wrote this book. Without floating, I'm certain that my life would be much darker, much more difficult, and far lonelier. Instead, I have discovered a freedom and self-confidence that I thought for a long time was gone forever. My relationships are thriving, and my career is fulfilling.

I believe this kind of transformation and recovery from mental illness is possible for you, too. But there was a time when I couldn't see how I would ever escape the darkness of anxiety and depression.

When my mental health was at its worst ten years ago, I was living in Los Angeles and growing worse and worse by the day. After suffering through a breakdown and my first panic attack on a business trip, I eventually found floating.

What I haven't told you is that I went through some twists and turns on my way there—sidetracks and so-called solutions that I think a number of people like me have tried. Maybe you can relate.

LETTING THE UNIVERSE STEP IN

I was still living in the heart of the Hollywood ghetto, not the sanest place to be. I remember seeing a billboard that said something about saving yourself and listed an address on Sunset Boulevard. For some desperate reason, I felt the need to reach out.

That's how I ended up attending a Scientology lunch meeting.

As I looked around, everyone was totally blank. It's like I was in a crowd of zombies. People would smile and say very normal things but in a very abnormal tone.

The therapy they suggested for my anxiety was equally as weird. I walked into a room with a counselor for my first session. I grabbed two cold metal rods that were supposed to measure something. The counselor had me talk through my entire breakdown over and over and over. In fact I closed my eyes sometime after lunch and didn't open them again until it was dark. I remember being in a trance of explanation and repetition.

Once I was done I did feel relief. In fact, that night I remember not having anxiety at all. I felt cured. Little did I know I was just mentally exhausted and unable to even think.

When I woke up the next morning, my mind was sieged with anxious thoughts. I definitely did not feel cured. I felt certifiably crazy.

To make matters worse, I couldn't believe I'd spent the whole day in a Scientologist church with weird people doing a weird therapy.

What's funny about that now is the empathy I feel for people who think floating is a weird therapy with weird people. Of course, the difference that I can explain to them is that I've found lasting benefits through my floating habit and authentic relationships in the floating community.

But a decade ago, before I had found a solution to my spiraling panic, I feared for my sanity. Surely this was the process psychotic people went through—joining an extremist church, doing weird rituals. I expected to have a complete breakdown at any moment.

Then one day I was driving in my car and my mother called. After some chitchat, she asked me if I was okay. I snapped and started balling. Then it all came tumbling out, everything I had been holding in and trying to hide from the people still left in my life. I was not okay. I was so far from okay. I thought I was going to die at any moment. My world and anything that made me happy had vanished. I was barely holding on.

My mother immediately assured me I would be fine, and she booked a flight for me back home to Utah. I threw some clothes in a bag and headed out.

When I got to the airport in L.A., I couldn't breathe. I just knew my last moment of duct-taped-together sanity was going to come apart in shreds in front of everyone before I could even make it home. I put on headphones and proceeded to try and calm myself. I breathed deeply, closed my eyes, and told myself, "Keep it together."

My mother picked me up in Utah. Being with her made things seem okay. Almost like I was the same old person I was before I left. There was something very comforting about being home. At the same time, it was stressful.

One of the worst aspects of going through mental problems is that you have to put the people you love through the same pain you're experiencing. You have moments of joy and it gives them hope, only to feel yourself sink down again and scare them. Throughout my recovery, I've had moments of "not wanting to go on anymore." When I would bring it up with people I cared about, I could see it terrified them. The last thing I wanted to do was scare them, but at times I needed them to know just how serious things were.

As we drove along the highway in Utah, I remember the sun streaming in through the car windows, and a part of me felt normal again. The other part dreaded the moment my mom had to see the real me.

"I GAVE UP CONTROL AND LET THE UNIVERSE STEP IN. FROM THERE, THINGS GOT BETTER."

We arrived at my grandparents' house. My mother had clued them in on our phone call. I remember the look of concern on their faces as they opened the door and hugged me. My uncle had succumbed to schizophrenia at the age of 18, so my grandparents had already lost a son to mental illness. They were scared of losing me too.

Grandparents' houses are always calm and peaceful, aren't they? As if the long years and old furniture shape the mood in the home. I felt like I was in a safe place. I lay down on the couch and looked at the spackled ceiling as I told my family about my breakdown, my lack of control, my constant fear, and my belief that I was going insane. They cried as they watched me.

As I lay there venting, I began to cry as well. I had the surreal feeling that I was on my deathbed. I felt like I had finally accepted the truth: I was indeed crazy. And in that moment, I felt myself give up.

It was over, and that was okay.

A sense of peace came over me, almost like I was infused with a divine spirit. As I felt it flood in, I heard the words of encouragement coming from my mom, my grandma, and grandpa. Things like "You're fine," "This is different from your uncle," and "You're not crazy."

Although I know this story sounds almost crazier

than what I had been going through, as I lay there on the couch surrounded by the people I loved, I fully relinquished control. It was as if I had passed through my own death, I had given up, and in that moment, I was saved.

I was saved by whatever you believe I was saved by. By whatever energy came in and filled me up. I will let you interpret what saved me. For me, the most natural interpretation is that I gave up control and let the universe step in.

From there, things got better.

THE STATE OF ANXIETY

The state of anxiety is something I am very familiar with. It's the prison of the mind where it feels as if everything is going to collapse. Where it feels as if one wrong move or decision could bring your life crashing down. The person you believe you are is hanging by a thread.

Anxiety disorders are the most common mental illness in the United States, affecting an estimated 40 million adults age 18 and older. That's 18 percent of the population.[12] From social anxiety and phobias to panic disorder and the closely related post-traumatic stress disorder, anxiety cripples its sufferers and destroys lives.

Experts believe that anxiety develops from a complex set of risk factors. Genetics, brain chemistry, personality, and life events may all play a part in why one person is prone to anxiety and another is not.[13]

But the sad truth is that only about one-third of us

will receive treatment.[14] In my case, my family helped me get some professional therapy, and I began to take medication to slow the onset of panic attacks. But it only helped to a point.

Over the years, anxiety prevented me from taking care of myself. I found myself eating and drinking not to nourish my body but to satisfy my brain's craving for a pleasurable experience to outweigh the constant state of fear. I didn't sleep—a common symptom of anxiety disorders. And I lost out on spending time with friends and family, traveling, and enjoying hobbies. For many people, these experiences are what make life worth living.

Most people with anxiety disorders suffer similar isolation and often share the same fears. Maybe some of these will sound familiar to you.

I have feared:
- Losing my mind
- Frightening and disappointing my loved ones
- Having to be hospitalized
- Burdening my family
- Suffering a worse breakdown and never being the same again
- Becoming known as a mentally unstable person
- Being treated differently and excluded from the lives of friends and family
- Experiencing fear in normal situations no matter what I do
- Having to take medication for the rest of my life
- Wondering if it's really me I'm experiencing or

just some weird medicated version of me
- Worrying myself into a state of utter isolation
- Missing my calling in life because I couldn't get it together
- Being weak and unable to handle people or situations without help
- Becoming dependent on alcohol or other substances that ease the anxiety temporarily
- And missing some solution that could change how I feel and finally free me.

I know those who suffer from anxiety aren't the only ones who feel these fears. Depression and PTSD often cause similar worries.

Dr. Rod Borrie, who has conducted float research on everything from anxiety to pain reduction, says, "Anxiety is about jumping into the future and painting all kinds of disasters."

He's right. Anxiety has caused me to dwell on scenarios that have never come to pass. But that fact alone isn't enough to stop the worrying, the obsessions, and the fear.

"Some of the self-healing we need to do mentally has to do with getting unstuck," Rod says.

WHEN ANXIETY TURNS TO PANIC

When someone with anxiety is stuck in that loop of fear and worry, it triggers feelings in the body like an elevated heart rate, sweating, and difficulty breathing that can spur even scarier thoughts. This is the beginning of a panic attack.

About 6 million people in the United States experience panic disorder each year. A more severe form of mental illness than generalized anxiety disorder, panic usually arises in early adulthood. Left untreated, recurring panic attacks usually worsen over time and can develop into agoraphobia—the fear of public places.[15]

I was well on my way to this lonely condition. When I worried about going insane from all the anxious thoughts in my head, I'd feel tightness in my chest that made me wonder if I was having a panic attack or a heart attack. This level of fear would make my hands start to shake. Looking at my hands, I'd become convinced that something was seriously wrong. My face would contort and if someone saw me, the shame of the situation would be overwhelming. My flight or fight response would kick in and the next thing I knew I'd be running out of the building or into the bathroom to pop a pill just to breathe.

On any given day, I was moments away from a trip to the mental ward and possibly, the collapse of my life.

In hindsight, as I write this book, I know it all sounds ridiculous to someone who has never experienced this kind of crippling mental illness. But this was daily life for me and others like me.

THE STATE OF FLOAT

When I first started floating these were the cycles I was battling. I was in a constant state of either fight or flight—or the fear of entering that state.

Everyone floats for the first time with different

expectations. I expected to love it. Turns out, I did love it right away. But that's not everyone's experience.

"THE STATE OF FLOAT IS LIKE A JOURNEY TO ANOTHER PLACE."

Most people hop into the tank very excited. They've usually seen videos and testimonials from floaters, and they're pretty enthusiastic about having their own experience. But no matter how they feel going in, I've found that more that 75 percent of the time, they come out of their first float and say, "It was okay. I liked the floating feeling." Or they might say, "It was hard getting comfortable" or "I got salt in my eyes." They rarely say, "I loved it!"

This is because the float tank, however nice and peaceful it might look, offers an experience that our bodies tell us is scary. You're getting in a tank filled with water, and the normal reaction is to fear drowning. You close the lid and the space gets smaller like you're stuck in a claustrophobic trap. Without sight, sound, or gravity to tell your mind which way is up, it's hard to predict what's coming—even though nothing is coming. But your brain and body kick into very natural responses, including tension. No wonder it's hard to relax!

People with anxiety have trouble overcoming those first couple of float reactions in order to get to the good stuff. This is why I tell people to float at least three times before making up their mind if it's right for them.

*Visit TalesFromTheTank.com to watch video testimonials on floating.

With a little self-coaching, you can convince yourself that it's safe and peaceful, and you'll begin to relax.

So much of anxiety consists of obsessive and compulsive thoughts. From my first float, I was amazed to discover that I could break the cycle and calm myself. I could focus on something positive and present. I discovered that not only had I built a meditation machine, I had built an anxiety reducing machine. It started to change everything in my life.

Rod Borrie's and Peter Suedfeld's research in the '90's showed that floating reduces agitation and phobic symptoms, as well as improving symptoms of insomnia.[16] It's the perfect anti-anxiety solution.

But I did have to put in some effort to turn down my thoughts or get "unstuck," as Rod says. In my early days in the float tank, I began visualizing my breathing or counted backwards from one hundred—discovering some of the techniques for meditation I've shared with you in the previous chapter. I used these simple visualizations to turn down my thinking and get into the most peaceful state possible. My goal was less and less brain function.

For me, the state of float is like a journey to another place.

Ultimately, I achieved that state, where I was simply feeling. I wasn't analyzing, prepping, computing, or observing. I was just feeling and being. This is the state that I really enjoy, and I must admit it is not easy to achieve. I have had moments in the tank of pure ecstasy. Some of the altered states I've reached in a tank have been amazing, and I can remember them in detail.

This turned-down state is the kryptonite to anxiety and panic. It is the exact opposite use of your brain and body. Rather than rapid-fire discomfort, it is calming, slow, and comfortable. The more you float, the more your brain and body become accustomed to this new way of existing.

YOUR BRAIN ON FLOATING

One of the theories about why this happens is we have two pathways in our brains: one to monitor our external systems and one to monitor our internal systems. This internal pathway, called interoception, is the one we don't think about consciously. It's busy providing signals about our heart beating, blood pulsing through our veins, our immune system, respiration, and countless other functions that occur with the cooperation of our brain but without our awareness on a conscious level.

Justin Feinstein, director of the Laureate Institute for Brain Research Float Clinic and Research Center in Tulsa, Oklahoma, says the first time he talked to someone who had floated, he knew he was hearing something revolutionary.

It was 2013, and he was working in the neuroscience laboratory at California Institute of Technology. His primary research focus was anxiety. "One of the research assistants who shared an office with me at the time came to me—I believe it was a Monday—and over the weekend she had just had her first float. At the time I had never even heard of what a float tank was. And she proceeded to tell me over the next several hours, with great drama, how intense and powerful this first float was for her."

The research assistant said she felt connected to a part of herself that she didn't even know existed. For hours afterward, she felt liberated.

"I listened with great curiosity because she was describing something that I'd been interested in for almost my entire life in research. What she was describing to me was a concept that's known in the field as interoception."

Justin says all of the signals about the inner workings of our bodies come into our brains through a dedicated pathway. He had spent more than a decade researching this pathway. "And when she was describing her first float to me, it became clear, even though she didn't use those words, that what she was accessing was her interoceptive self."

What intrigued Justin most was the coincidence of hearing about this access to the interoceptive self soon after he had learned that a disruption to this pathway was a common denominator in people who suffered from anxiety.

"So there's something about this interoceptive pathway that's critical for anxiety," Justin says. "It seems to be dysregulated in anxiety disorders, and when you float, it provides sort of a sneak peek into this pathway in a way that you could never access outside of a float."

Justin floated for the first time soon after this, and he

was hooked. Not only is it a practice he's incorporated into his own life, it's the major focus of his research. He now works with Dr. Martin Paulus at LIBR to study, among other benefits, how floating targets the interoceptive system.

And how it frees countless people from the prison of anxiety.

THE BLACK CLOUD OF DEPRESSION

Depression is one of the most misunderstood illnesses. People who are battling depression often are accused of being lazy, unmotivated, or simply pessimistic. Well-meaning friends and family might tell someone who is depressed to "snap out of it," "just get off the couch and get moving," or "look on the bright side." None of this advice is inherently bad, but for a depressed person, it is irrelevant and ineffective.

"APERSONWHONEEDSGLASSESCANNOT WILLHERSELFTOSEEBETTERANYMORE THANAPERSONWITHDEPRESSIONCANWILL HIMSELF TO BE HAPPY."

Major Depressive Disorder is the leading cause of disability for ages 15 to 44 in the United States. In a given year, 18 million adults are affected by some form of depression, which also adversely affects other chronic conditions like asthma, arthritis, cancer, diabetes, and cardiovascular disease.[17]

You can think of depression like quicksand. You sink deeper and deeper despite your best efforts to get yourself out in standard ways. All the exercise in the world sometimes isn't enough to lift someone's mood. Happy events, positive feedback, and support from loved ones are all well and good, but depression often worsens despite outside circumstances.

What depression does seem to respond to is work that we do on the inside.

I believe we have the ability to impact just about everything in life, but not always in the way we want. A person who needs glasses cannot will herself to see better any more than a person with depression can will himself to be happy.

Over the last decade, in my own search for answers, I've studied the way depression manifests and how it is treated. It seems to have two aspects: the part you can control with thought, and the part you can't.

As someone who believes in the power of positive thinking and attitude being at the heart of so much in this world, it was incredibly tough for me to admit that my depressive thoughts were out of my control.

After starting therapy and medication back home in Utah, I felt some relief but still had the sinking feeling that medication was for lazy people. Even as I struggled with depression myself, I fell prey to the stereotypes about this illness. But the truth was although I was motivated to work and live an active life, no matter what I did, I couldn't shake the dark cloud and depressed thoughts that would roll into my life every morning upon waking.

I would go to the gym and get temporary relief through the release of endorphins but it would fade. I would try to do something I used to love, like skateboarding, but it didn't hold my interest. Everything I tried would offer a glimmer of hope, but it wasn't lasting.

Fortunately, medication allowed me to see some improvement long enough to seek more natural solutions that did offer long-term relief—like floating.

A WORD ABOUT MEDICATION

Before we move on, let me just say something about medication. Taking a pill without doing any other work to fix the source of your problem is a waste of time, in my opinion. I often think of this in a physical way for comparison.

Let's say I was overweight because I didn't maintain healthy habits. Years before, maybe I injured my back and that's why I avoid exercise. Well, if I finally find a medication that relieves my back pain and the side effects don't prevent me from rigorous exercise, wouldn't you expect me to start hitting the gym a few days a week? Or walking around the block? Or at least taking the stairs at work?

But what if I didn't do anything differently—instead, chose to stay on the couch and continue to gain weight and jeopardize my health?

The pain medication would be merely a temporary escape from unrelenting symptoms that are clearly going to worsen over time—requiring me to take more and more medication to achieve the same relief.

I think this is very similar to someone in a depressive state that results in unhealthy habits, broken relationships, and frustrated dreams. Taking medication in hopes that all of these things will get better simply because you have a temporary fix for your mood is unrealistic.

However, taking medication so you can get out of bed in the morning, feel motivated to walk daily, get to your therapist appointment, and start taking care of your personal issues is a very different situation.

Healing takes work. A problem can only be solved at its source.

When I hear people balk at the idea of taking an anti-depressant, I'm sad for them. What about our friend who has poor vision and finds herself needing glasses? Some people are born with physical disabilities and will need help no matter what they do. Glasses are not "natural," and she will need them for life. They're a great option in our modern society. For many people this may be their reality with medication.

This approach worked for me. I hope, if you or someone you love is struggling with depression—or anxiety or any other mental illness—you'll consider using medication in combination with a healthy regimen of other solutions. It can truly be a temporary avenue to deeper healing when used properly.

NATURAL SOLUTIONS TO DEPRESSION OR ANXIETY

Floating can play a huge part in depression recovery and happiness maintenance, but I want to acknowledge that there are many more pieces involved. Finding natural solutions to depression or anxiety gives you a real sense of independence, so I always encourage people to take control and discover some of these solutions for themselves. But I do want to note that natural solutions alone are not always enough to truly treat depression and severe anxiety.

With that said, I'd like to tell you about some methods I've used to improve my mental health.

Eating Healthy—I've tried it all when it comes to nutrition: eating without rules and gaining weight, counting calories and just eating smaller portions of the same junk, and super-restrictive diets that are painful and inconvenient. Lately, here's what I've come up with that's working for me now. First, spikes in blood sugar seem to be the main source of weight gain and food addiction in the United States. If you want to see more on why and how this may be happening in your own diet, I suggest watching the documentary *Fed Up*. Second, worry about nutrition not calories. But overall remember that nobody else's answer for eating healthy should be yours. Find your own path.

Staying Fit—Doing a little bit every day is more powerful than doing a ton a couple times a week. What can you reasonably get yourself to do every day? Maybe it's morning pushups, taking the stairs, parking far away, taking daily walks, or finding an active hobby. You're much more likely to keep at it if you enjoy it. I do sixty pushups and ten pull-ups before every shower, and I've gotten more results with this low-stress method than when I went to the gym three days a week and beat myself up physically. Small, healthy habits compound over time to give you big results.

Healthy Relationships—There's a saying that has changed my life in many ways: "You are the average of the five people you spend the most time with." You can be the strongest willed person on earth, but if you hang around with negative, toxic people, you will soak up some of their attitude. Put strict limits on the amount of time you spend with negative people and try to keep the conversation and interactions as healthy as possible. Seek examples among loved ones for what a healthy relationship looks like or ask advice from a counselor. Think of it as using a personal trainer for your relationships.

Healthy Psychology—Your psychology is either where the magic happens or the inner hell is constructed. I value my mental health so much that I would trade all other good things in life for it, hands down. There is nothing quite as scary as being in a mental prison that you can't escape. I've spent more than 500 hours in the chair learning about my psychology—the best time and money I've ever spent. Don't get me wrong: Not all psychological health requires time in a therapist's chair. Much of it can be done on your own with a teacher, mentor, or friend.

Fun and Enjoyment—Do the things you love regularly and don't work yourself to death. If you have vacation guilt or can't take a day off, believe me, it's affecting your mental health. It's okay to take time for yourself.

Check out the book *Play It Away* by Charlie Hoehn for more on this. It's an awesome read!

Meditation, Reflection, Introspection—Although this can be done outside of a tank, floating is, of course, ideal for this practice. But whether you use a tank or not, be sure you regularly create quiet space for yourself. It's vital to your mental health.

Floating—Flotation has been shown to have a similarly beneficial effect on the symptoms of depression as on anxiety. A study in Sweden showed that participants exhibited lowered blood pressure, reduced anxiety, depression, stress, and negative outlook. But they also showed an increase in overall optimism, energy, and positive outlook.[18] What this shows is that not only does floating help alleviate depression, but it also helps the floater start creating a new, more positive and hopeful mindset.

Rod believes this may be due to the fact that when we float, we're forced to live fully in the moment rather than dwelling on past pains. "The research shows that people have an increased feeling of well-being," he says. "You're more relaxed. You come so much into the present. You're not digging around and rehashing old regrets and losses."

LIVING WITH PTSD

In this age of ongoing strife and violence, chances are that you know someone with post-traumatic stress disorder. Occurring in some people who have experienced traumatic or life-threatening events, PTSD can be debilitating due to the accompanying depression, anxiety, and physical symptoms, which often last for years if left untreated. It's estimated that 7.7 million Americans age 18 and older suffer from PTSD.[19]

I'd like to tell you about one of them.

When he was 21 years old, Michael Harding enlisted in the Australian Army, and in 2010 he was deployed to Afghanistan with the 6th Battalion of the Royal Australian Regiment. During his tour, Michael was involved in a firefight that lasted three and a half hours and resulted in the death of his section second-in-command.

Michael soon began experiencing full body twitches. He was evacuated and diagnosed with Conversion Disorder, a form of PTSD with functional neurological symptoms. He received a medical discharge in 2012 and returned home to his wife Bek a different man.

"Michael was a very confident person prior to the Army," Bek says. "He was the life of the party, loved to go out, had a massive group of friends. And the minute he came back from Afghanistan, that all changed."

Back at home, Michael received treatment from veterans' services that included exposure therapy, cognitive behavioral therapy, and a number of different medications.

"They only exacerbated everything," Michael says. "Made my condition worse. The medication suppressed everything, and because I couldn't really feel anything emotionally, I was a zombie and wouldn't get out of bed before twelve."

Bek says the medication kept Michael from feeling,

which prevented him from working through his trauma. "You can't process what you've experienced," she says. "You can't even experience happiness when you're on as much as what Michael was on. There were times when he'd be getting really worked up and he'd say to me, 'I really need to cry but I physically cannot.' I was like, that's not right. That's not a human response. That's not normal at all."

Feeling more and more hopeless, Michael turned to alcohol. "I was just a mess," he says. "Bek would have to pick me up from car parks, lying in the gutter with spew on myself or come around and pick me up from a mate's place where I was unable to get out of the chair."

Bek calls this time "the lowest of lows." She says he would enter dissociative states where he would shut down mentally and be unable to function. He couldn't cook or drive or do most of the daily requirements for living. Bek had to quit her full-time job and take over his care almost completely.

"The psychological, emotional, and mental toll it took on me was dramatic as well," Bek says. "There were basically two very unwell people living together." At one point, Bek's own therapist suggested she be admitted to a psychiatric facility for treatment.

She became desperate to try something else to help Michael recover. They started with nutrition, doing a juice cleanse that helped Michael lose about 30 of the 80 pounds he had gained since his discharge. After the initial cleanse, they focused on eating a plant-based, whole-food diet. They also tried medical cannabis, which is illegal in Australia, but they were willing to try anything and had read the studies being done in the United States about positive impacts.

The combination of these approaches, plus daily exercise, inspired Michael to get off all medication. And he saw some progress. "Things were going all right, but I was still having a lot of night sweats and nightmares, and my twitches would still occur. I had a lot of social anxiety," he says.

Michael had returned to his job when he got home, but he only lasted four months. No one else would hire him. He avoided large crowds and even family gatherings. He disconnected from his civilian friends, and most of his Army buddies didn't understand what he was going through—although sadly, a few of them later learned firsthand as they had their own experiences with PTSD.

One day while Bek was researching alternative therapies online, she came across a video of Joe Rogan, former host of *Fear Factor*, talking about floating. She watched a few more videos, looked up research on REST and its positive effects on anxiety and depression, and knew it would be great for PTSD as well.

But Michael was tough to convince. He had begun work with some volunteer organizations, trying to help fellow vets in their struggle to regain a normal life back home. After six months and Bek's promise to pay for the float, Michael gave in. He was only one week away from having to speak at a fundraiser for an event he had helped organize, so his symptoms were worsening with his stress level.

"I was quite skeptical going along for the first one," he says. "I was like, oh man, it's just some salty bath I could just do this at home."

The float center was over an hour away from their house, but the technician was patient and knowledgeable, putting Michael at ease. He recommended that Michael try three sessions all in that first week.

After one hour in the tank, Michael was hooked. "I hopped out feeling on top of the world." With a big grin on his face, he gave Bek a kiss and said, "Let's book the next two!"

"I was converted as soon as I tried it," he says.

His third session was on Friday, the day of the fundraiser. "I still had a lot of anxiety because it was probably about 150-odd people at the event, but it was a lot more maintainable. I was able to participate and help coordinate people."

Bek spent her time talking with veterans and attendees, telling them about their successes with natural and alternative therapies for PTSD. As she was explaining their newest adventure with floating to a friend, she heard something that brought tears to her eyes.

Michael was speaking. Into a microphone. In front of 150 people.

"I balled my eyes out," Bek says. "It was the biggest turnaround because I honestly thought during the week that he wasn't even going to be able to make it to the event. He was that worked up and stressed out, and a lot of his symptoms had returned. So then to hear him get up and talk on the microphone, I instantly broke into tears.

It was even bigger and better than what I ever imagined. It was incredible."

Both Bek and Michael floated twice a week for the next six months. Then they purchased a reconditioned tank and set it up at home so they could float as often as they like.

Today, combining a floating habit with healthy eating, exercise, meditation, yoga, medical cannabis, positive affirmations, and peer-to-peer-rehabilitation, Michael has finally found his way back to a life he loves. He's become an advocate for the use of Integrative Therapies in the treatment of PTSD and other mental health issues. He serves as a mentor in Trojan's Trek, a peer-to-peer rehab program for veterans in South Australia, and speaks publicly as an active member in other ex-service organizations and charities.

FLOATING FOR PTSD RELIEF

When I spoke with Michael, I was struck by how many opportunities there are for people suffering from PTSD to find freedom and healing through floating.

Anthony Natale, a veteran counselor, writer, and massage therapist, suffered from PTSD for years that caused him horrible anxiety and insomnia. After his first float, he slept through the entire night, and he knew he'd found the answer to his years of struggle. Today, Anthony is on a mission to expand the uses of the float tank for developing and enhancing human potential.

Anthony compares floating to cleaning out your computer hard drive. "Sometimes people can go to the mountains and get away or something like that." But this doesn't always make much difference in anxiety or PTSD, he says, "Because you've still got to come back into your regular life. With floating, the sensory deprivation time is kind of like a defragging of the hard drive. What floating does really effectively is clean out and upgrade, so when you go back in the same situation, you're using different aspects of your nervous system that maybe weren't available to you at first. They are available to you post-float and can be used to make a lot of changes."

Essentially, Anthony says that you come back to your regular reality with more capability and more processing power. As a result, he says your brain is faster, more efficient, and more focused.

Floating is everything I believe a person with anxiety, depression, or PTSD should be striving for. I've come to love having a state that is familiar to me other than anxiety. I've changed the way I feel, think, and react permanently. It's like riding a bike: When I need that peaceful state, I can remember it and draw it out.

Everyone battling mental illness should be floating. It's an amazing environment for working out negative thought patterns and cycles, and for training your body in how to behave and feel. It has returned me to my life—it has given me a life. And a beautiful one, at that.

TO KEEP THE BODY
IN GOOD HEALTH IS
ADUTY...OTHERWISE
WE SHALL NOT BE
ABLE TO KEEP OUR
MIND STRONG AND
CLEAR.
-BUDDHA

CHAPTER 4
RELIEVE PHYSICAL PAIN AND OPTIMIZE PERFORMANCE

Our brains and bodies are part of one incredible system. It's easy to forget that what impacts one also impacts the other. But when your body interferes with your ability to think, feel, and live to your highest potential, this mind-body link becomes all too clear.

From men and women suffering with chronic pain to professional athletes, millions of people spend much of their day focused on their physical well-being. They seek pain relief and performance optimization through traditional medicine, prescription drugs, and alternative therapies.

The breakthrough that so many have discovered in recent years is the immense and sometimes immediate effect of floating.

In this chapter, I want to share some stories of people who found both relief and rejuvenation through floating, professional athletes who use floating on a regular basis to enhance their performance, and experts who have witnessed remarkable physical benefits from floating routines.

PAIN RELIEF

All of us have experienced pain whether in the form of injury or a chronic condition. Pain is the leading cause of emergency room visits, and significant or chronic pain affects more Americans than diabetes, heart disease, and cancer combined.[20]

Treatment varies according to the type, intensity, and duration of the pain, but there are some common treatments that most people pursue. Let's break them down into the major categories.

Alternative treatments—Acupuncture, massage, and yoga are considered alternative treatments for pain. These activities are intended to improve circulation, alleviate pain, and improve muscle tone. People often use alternative methods in combination with more traditional treatments.

Chiropractic care—A professional chiropractor can be consulted to alleviate back pain, but the spinal adjustment process might also assist with other sources of pain.

Physical therapy—Ideal for pain that results from injury or surgical procedures, physical therapy comes in many forms. Heat, ultrasound, electrical stimulation, and muscle release techniques all offer distinct benefits to muscles and soft tissues. Supervised exercises increase flexibility, strengthen muscles, and improve posture.

Surgery—Chronic pain due to musculoskeletal issues, as well as nerve damage, might benefit from surgery. However, surgery often is a last resort when other treatments have ceased to provide any benefit.

OTC medication—From pain relievers such as acetaminophen to nonsteroidal anti-inflammatory drugs (NSAIDs) such as ibuprofen or naproxen sodium, there are multiple options for over-the-counter (OTC) treatment of pain. But these medications also can come with detrimental side effects. NSAIDs can raise blood pressure, increase the risk of heart disease, produce ulcers or gastrointestinal bleeding, and cause kidney damage. Acetaminophen is easier on the stomach but can cause liver damage with regular use of even small doses.[21] Over-the-counter topical ointments and salves also might provide some relief.

Prescription medication—For injuries and chronic soft tissue pain, physicians may prescribe muscle relaxants to help patients reduce tension and therefore pain in the affected muscles. Injections of cortisone, an anti-inflammatory drug, are used to decrease nerve pain. Lately, doctors have been prescribing antidepressants for pain, even when depression isn't an issue. Studies have shown that tricyclic antidepressants have a positive benefit when used for chronic pain from arthritis to nerve damage to back pain.[22] However, some patients have a problem with the side effects these medications produce, especially when there is no depression to be treated.

Of course, narcotics are the strongest medical weapon against pain. Opioids such as codeine, hydrocodone, and oxycodone are a few of the most commonly prescribed drugs for acute or chronic pain that is unresponsive to other treatments. But long-term use of these narcotics can lead to dependence and other dangerous side effects.[23] Sadly, this dependence leads to misuse and even death. Unintentional overdose deaths involving prescription opioids have quadrupled since 1999 and outnumber those from cocaine and heroin combined.[24]

While all of these options have their place in the treatment of injury and chronic pain, I truly believe that floating might prove to be a universal pain reliever— one with no negative side effects and with benefits far beyond physical well-being.

FLOATING TO RELIEVE PAIN FROM INJURY

I used to work out at the gym a few times a week, and then I'd hit a wall with my motivation. I'd get sick of the immense effort, the huge time commitment, and the minimal results. So I'd start slacking on my exercise habit. Then, feeling guilty, I'd hit it hard again one day. Inevitably, this kind of on again, off again routine resulted in muscle strains. I'm lucky it wasn't worse.

Whether you've been injured through exercise, physical labor, an accident, or some other situation in your life, injuries can linger and threaten your peace of mind.

Floating has been shown to reduce pain from mild injuries such as muscle strains.[25]

Ashkahn Jahromi, co-founder of Float On in Portland, Oregon, and co-creator of the annual Float Conference, says that some of the most profound results he sees coming out of float tanks at their center involve physical pain. "People come out saying that their shoulders haven't been relaxed in twelve years, or they haven't *not* had aches for years. The relief is so evident."

Ashkahn tells the story of a previous employee at the 24-hour float center who was a piano player: "He would work our night shift, and he would float afterwards early in the morning. He said that floating all the time made him realize that his whole body was starting to twist to the right a little bit from playing the piano. With such a focus on his right hand, he just spent a lot of his floats trying to re-align his body and stop the rotation from happening.

"You know, you get really used to how your body feels, and if your shoulder is kind of aching or whatever, it just becomes normal for you and you forget about it, in a certain sense. It just becomes the status quo. Then you hop into a float tank and you don't feel it for a little bit. That puts a spotlight on the different things in your body that maybe you should be paying attention to, and maybe that you should be trying to work on."

CHRONIC PAIN

For more than 100 million Americans, pain is something they are very aware of on a daily basis.[26] These chronic pain sufferers might understand the source of their distress, but many are confused or frustrated by how to treat it. They've likely been through several—if not all—of the treatment options I listed above. Years of struggle, financial strain, and emotional turmoil take an incredible toll on victims of chronic pain.

Chronic pain is caused by a number of conditions. Some of the most common we see in our own customers are arthritis, back pain, migraine headaches, and fibromyalgia.

Studies have shown that REST (floating) reduces stiffness, muscle spasms, and joint pain in rheumatoid arthritis sufferers.[27]

Headache patients in a flotation study reported reduced frequency, intensity, and duration of headaches by up to 57 percent after six months of floating.[28]

As the owner of NOLA Float Tanks, Spencer Fossier has used floating for years to treat back pain he says was caused by sitting for extended periods of time. "I feel like my back pain stems from being compressed," he says. "Sitting down for so long, you place all that weight stacked up on your spine. It's pressure all the way down from your head through your waist. That can actually shorten people."

When floating, the back can decompress thanks to a lack of gravity and the total relaxation of the muscles around the spine.

"All of a sudden we have a 90 percent reduction in gravity's forces on your body," says Anthony Natale, a veteran counselor and massage therapist who speaks on floating's benefits. "You get an inch-and-a-half of spinal decompression."

For people with back pain or injury, this decompression can result in both an immediate and lasting relief from pain and discomfort.

"IHADTWOWHOLECOMPLETELYPAINFREE DAYSAFTERMYFIRST90-MINUTEFLOATAT A FLOAT CENTER."

"I think floating helps reassemble my body," Spencer says. "My muscles aren't necessarily forced to assume one shape or the other, as at a desk or on the couch. When I'm floating, my body has the ability to just let go and express itself how it should be."

Dr. Rod Borrie, who has researched the positive impact of floating since the '70s, leads the general population study called The Fibromyalgia Flotation Project (FFP). The international, voluntary project was created to study the efficacy of REST as a treatment for fibromyalgia and was organized by the International Flotation Research Group.

Early research points to the effectiveness of floating in relieving fibromyalgia and other chronic pain. In one study, every test patient experienced a reduction in the intensity of their pain.[29]

The first study reported by the FFP in 2012 provided evidence that flotation does in fact improve the lives of people with fibromyalgia by decreasing their pain, muscle tension, anxiety, and stress. It also increases their freedom of movement, energy, mood, and quality of sleep. Most of these improvements continued as long as the patients kept up with regular float sessions.[30]

In research since then, Rod has found that, "If you can get someone with chronic pain to float on a regular basis, you can reduce the amount of medication they're taking significantly."

This is a huge claim, but Lynn Taylor, one familiar with Rod's study and a client of my company Zen Float Co, has found this to be true in her own life. Before floating, Lynn was dependent on daily doses of anti-inflammatory and pain medications.

"If I wasn't taking the ibuprofen, I probably wouldn't have been walking around," she says. Most days, she limped out of bed, instantly in pain upon waking. When OTC medications stopped working, she was given a prescription NSAID, which she says was only effective for about six months.

"I started on these rounds of different drugs that I was not happy with," she says. "I decided I'd look for something that wasn't going to cause me bad side effects."

Lynn came across floating through an old friend, who had opened a float center. When she read that the practice could have an impact on her fibromyalgia symptoms, she says, "My eyes literally filled with tears. Sometimes you just have a moment in time when you intuitively know that you have found the key to change your life."

Soon after, she joined the FFP. But the closest float center was two hours away from her home. During her research into floating, she came across our original Kickstarter campaign for the Zen Float Tent. We were still getting things going, and Lynn was one of our first customers.

Before she ordered her float tent, we recommended

that she try a commercial float to be sure she liked it and that it would work for her condition.

"I had two whole completely pain free days after my first 90-minute float at a float center," Lynn says. That's all the convincing she needed.

Today, she floats at home regularly. "I discovered that I am a night floater. I've had considerable trouble in the past few years falling asleep because it's just so hard to get my muscles to relax. I go straight to bed after my float and fall asleep within five to ten minutes. It's really nice for my husband as well, no more keeping him awake as he has to be an early riser for work. The sleep I have after a float is deep and comfortable. My husband says I used to roll over and moan in pain in my sleep. No more of that, either."

Floating has also augmented the other treatments that Lynn uses for her fibromyalgia symptoms, including muscle stiffness and back pain. Floating before stretching or yoga classes has increased her range of motion and decreased post-workout soreness. She also floats before seeing her chiropractor, who has seen measurable differences in the effectiveness of her adjustments after a float session in comparison to when she used to come in without floating. Today, instead of going every three weeks for an adjustment, she has stretched that to four weeks and hopes to keep adding time between appointments.

Although Lynn says that some of the results seem like common sense, she believes the float tank's unique environment has been "like magic" to her improved well-being and pain reduction. "It is nothing new that warm water and Epsom salts are going to ease aches and pains," she says, "but floating really goes so much further than that. Adding the other components of complete quiet and darkness, along with the feeling of total weightlessness allows both your body and your mind to fully relax."

Lynn no longer takes any pain medication, not even OTC pills. She does limit her physical exertion, but she says, "If I stick to a reasonable lifestyle, I can live in comfort once again."

OPTIMIZING ATHLETIC PERFORMANCE

If floating can relieve pain, doesn't it just make sense that it can also optimize physical performance? For decades now, athletes all over the world have been using float tanks to enhance muscle repair, aid visualization, and sharpen mental states.

Here are a few of the professional athletes and teams that have reported using floating as a regular part of their training and recovery regimens:

- NFL's Dallas Cowboys
- NFL's Philadelphia Eagles
- MLB's Arizona Diamondbacks
- Australian Institute of Sport for Olympic athletes
- Carl Lewis, Gold medal Olympian
- Swedish Olympic teams
- United Kingdom Olympic teams
- UFC's Pat Healy

Reportedly, top athletes have also chosen to have tanks installed in their homes, including Larry Fitzgerald of the Arizona Cardinals, Tom Brady of the New England Patriots, Marvin Jones of the Cincinnati Bengals, and Wayne Rooney of Manchester United. Former Texas Ranger Pete O'Brien opened @Peace Flotation Spa in Colleyville, Texas, after his retirement from baseball.

The relaxation benefits and stress reduction from floating are only one part why these athletes choose to use float tanks on a regular basis.

MUSCLE REPAIR

Strenuous and frequent workouts put strain on the body. Professional athletes routinely submit their bodies to unusual demands. Whether it's injury or soreness from intense practices, muscle pain and fatigue are a part of daily life for many of these elite performers.

Fortunately, as I've mentioned in previous chapters, float tanks increase endorphins, reducing pain. Floating also reduces cortisol levels, which are responsible for some of the negative effects of stress on the body. The reduction in cortisol, combined with the increase in endorphins makes for a powerful pain reliever.

In addition, floating increases blood circulation, enhancing the flushing of toxins from muscles and decreasing recovery time.

Epsom salts are known to reduce swelling and detoxify the system, but some experts even point to exposure to magnesium in the salt water as having a beneficial impact on muscle recovery. One study reported increased physical endurance, improved force and muscle metabolism.[31]

Of course, the lack of gravity takes pressure off the muscles, tissues, and joints, aiding in speedier recovery times and reduced pain. And the rejuvenating effect that people report after floating minimizes fatigue and optimizes athletic resilience.

All of this means that marathon runners are back on their feet faster, professional weight lifters are back in the gym sooner, and UFC fighters are back in fighting form quicker than without the help of a float tank.

In an interview with *The Washington Times*, Maurice Edu, a professional soccer player for the Philadelphia Union, said floating has made a difference in his performance: "I was kind of a little bit wary about it, but intrigued in the same breath. For me, I felt the benefit straight away. I think it helped me to recover between games a lot quicker."[32]

Ultra-marathon runner Yassine Diboun of Portland, Oregon, has become an avid floater. Running fifty to one hundred miles in a race would leave Yassine nearly crippled for two weeks afterward.

"Your joints hurt. Your muscles are fried. Your connective tissues are fried, and you're just kind of hobbling around like an old man," he says. Now, he finds that his recovery time is basically cut in half thanks to floating as part of his training.

"I think the benefits of floating are tremendous," he says. "I don't think people realize how beneficial it is to spend ninety minutes without having any pressure on your body. I always tell people, even if you have the most comfortable bed in the world at your home, when you go lie down in that bed, there's still pressure. There's still pressure from your skeletal frame pushing into the mattress. So when I go lay in the float tank and I'm just suspended on the surface of the water, I'm completely weightless and anti-gravity and there's no pressure against me. It feels very natural."

That's one of the things I love most about floating— and that others find so intriguing about it from the first time they float: It's natural. There's nothing super complicated about floating. No drugs. No complex procedures. It's a natural, easy way to boost your body's recovery and reduce pain.

VISUALIZATION

I have used a float tank successfully with visualization. But for athletes, this process can go a step further and enhance performance on a whole other level.

"IT'S AN AMAZING PHENOMENON THAT WE CAN TAKE ADVANTAGE OF DURING FLOTATION LIKE NEVER BEFORE."

Visualization is the rehearsal in your mind of something you need to perform in reality.

For me this was giving a speech. A few days before I was supposed to speak, I hopped in the tank. I went through my speech from the very beginning when I was sitting in the chair waiting to be called on stage. Because of the zero stimulus environment of the tank, it is much easier to get into your thoughts and not be distracted. I visualized getting up, walking on stage, and delivering the speech. I repeated that process, and I also went through possible scenarios like an interruption or a mistake.

It feels like the ultimate preparation when you know that nothing that can come up that you haven't been through before. In the tank I could even feel the uneasy feelings because my thoughts were more vivid. It was a type of exposure therapy to the discomfort of giving a speech.

This is very much the same process athletes go through while visualizing themselves executing the swing or the shot or the jump.

Brain studies show that thoughts produce the same mental instruction as the actions themselves. Mental imagery affects the same cognitive processes in the brain like perception, memory, and motor control.[33] The brain is training without the need of the body. It's an amazing phenomenon that we can take advantage of during flotation like never before.

Yassine has read the accounts by athletes like Carl Lewis who visualize their events beforehand, and he's chosen to use the float tank for visualization in addition to enhancing his physical recovery.

"For a lot of these long races, I break down the course and what I know is going to be coming at me," he says. "I'm literally thinking about the entire race, every aspect of it. What I do during the float is I picture everything in my mind – I mean from getting ready for the race, to going to the start line, seeing myself on the start line, almost like I'm a drone camera hovering above the whole start."

Yassine says there's a lot that goes into an ultra-marathon in terms of logistics, getting to aid stations, achieving certain milestones, pushing through mental and physical challenges at various points in the race. His float tank visualization is now key to his winning strategy.

MENTAL STATE

Whether it's the confidence you need going into an athletic endeavor or the ability to maintain your peak levels throughout the performance, your mental state is where it's at. Professional trainers also call this arousal regulation.

Arousal is the amount of energy you have throughout an event. It can be too low and show up as a lack of energy or alertness, or too high and result in the inability to stay calm and focused when pressures increase.

As I've talked about in previous chapters, floating can be used effectively to regulate the inability to stay calm and focused. Much like the way you can recall and practice a calm state when faced with anxiety, you can draw on the same practice to bring you down in an athletic event. It is a state you are familiar with and can enter on your own once you know how. For athletes in times of high pressure, this cognitive skill can prove priceless.

"I think floating gives me an advantage in a couple

different ways," Yassine says. But primary for him are "mental toughness and preparation."

Similar benefits have been found in the sport of free diving. Journalist James Nestor discovered free diving while on assignment for *Outside* magazine. He attended the 2011 Free Diving World Championships. "It's a very weird competition in which competitors challenge one another to see how deep they can dive on a single breath and come back conscious."

Unfortunately, not all of the competitors did come back conscious, and James was turned off by the competitive side of the sport with all its unnecessary risks. But he was intrigued by the practice. So much so that he ended up writing a book about it. In *Deep: Freediving, Renegade Science, and What the Ocean Tells Us about Ourselves*, James explores natural oceanic phenomena and human potential.

He says that free diving offers a kind of mental preparedness and confidence that's invaluable for athletes. In fact, over the last few years, Red Bull sent some of their sponsored Olympic athletes to a free diving camp in Hawaii to train.

"When you're a hundred feet down in the water and you can't take a sip of an oxygen tank or your lungs will explode, and no one can help you, you just learn to cope." The more you practice, the easier it becomes to cope with that stress, "with your body's physical reactions, with your mind telling you this is insane."

James says our modern world has us spoiled. "Everything's at our fingertips at all times. And we're accustomed to thinking that our body needs all these things constantly to function." But a hundred or two hundred years ago, he says we might go a few days without food or twelve hours without water if we were traveling, and our bodies are fine with that.

He says free diving "resets you and shows you about all of this lost human potential that we have. Your body's built to dive this deep and once you do it, you think wow, if I can do this, what else can I do?"

This type of confidence, along with the meditative power it requires to free dive responsibly, is similar to the effect of floating. And while free diving is his preference for getting in the zone, James doesn't always have the opportunity to dive. "So that's where floating comes in," he says.

"They are very similar in a lot of ways. With floating I can let go more than I can in free diving. ...

I use it creatively. It's been the biggest boom to me, even more so than meditation. Because inevitably I'll go into the float tank thinking about work, trying to remove it from my mind and then inevitably at the end of it, I'll have most of my work problems solved, stories written. I can just go home and write them down, because you're allowing the chatter in your mind to go away and allowing your brain to do what it wants to do.

For James, whose first love is the ocean, floating is the next best thing. "It makes life more enjoyable."

More and more, people are realizing that athletic potential is grounded in the brain and not just the body. One of the major benefits of floating is the enhancement of that mind-body connection. It allows athletes to see themselves as more than just physical instruments, but also as powerful mental performers who can increase their stamina and strength through their mental health as well as their physical training.

Floating is a natural, safe, and proven way to reduce pain, enhance physical recovery, and optimize athletic performance. As we learn more and more about the benefits of floating on the body, I know we'll see even more uses of this incredible journey to well-being.

WE ARE WHAT WE
REPEATEDLY DO.
EXCELLENCE, THEN,
IS NOT AN ACT, BUT A
HABIT.
-ARISTOTLE

CHAPTER 5
FIND YOUR FLOAT HABIT

Floating isn't the easiest thing to explain to people. When I first started floating, I worried about what my friends and family would think about a grown man hopping into a big tank of salt water and closing the lid.

I used to say, "It's a pitch black tank where you can't see, hear, or feel anything, and I'm using it to explore consciousness."

And that's true. But that much information sometimes puts people off if they have preconceived ideas about mind expansion. So now I just say, "It's a meditation environment."

I hope you realize by now that it's so much more than that.

The far-reaching effects of floating are still being researched. Studies continue around the world on floating's benefits for various mental health issues, medical conditions, and physical challenges.

"THE MORE YOU FLOAT, THE MORE BENEFITS YOU UNLOCK."

Already, REST has been shown to improve speech, learning, and overall behavioral and cognitive function in autistic children.[34] Another study documented behavioral improvements in Alzheimer's patients and better muscle control among cerebral palsy patients, as well as lower rates of relapse in people who were trying to reduce alcohol intake or lose weight.[35] And floating therapy has been shown to be an effective technique in smoking cessation.[36]

The future of floating is one filled with new applications, a more open acceptance among the public, and an expansion of what we're capable of as human beings. It's an exciting time to discover your own potential.

The fact is that the more you float, the more benefits you unlock, including mind expansion and spiritual exploration.

Yes, floating is a proven aid for mental health, physical well-being, and stress reduction, but it also touches something deeper inside of us. And before we move on to discuss how you can establish the best floating habit for your particular circumstances, I want to tell you a bit more about what might be in store for you down the line.

SPIRITUAL EXPLORATION

When I ask people why they want to float, the most common answer is some variation of spiritual exploration. It's a really big deal to people, yet it's hard to explain.

For me it was entering the space where I don't exist as a human. Where I forget about my body, my environment, my troubles, and just be. I suppose you could say I enter the state where I exist as spirit.

Anthony Natale says this is a common experience—and desire—among floaters. He's found that people are either looking for that deeper experience or are just content with the more immediate effects of floating on stress and physical health.

"That's the nice thing about floating," he says. "Everybody can get in the float tank and just have a great time. "

But some people feel compelled to float for hours at a time. "It's like a big wave surfer versus somebody who kind of goes out and plays on a boogie board," Anthony says, while describing surfers' need for big waves. "We're looking for something real, man. We want to go to the edge and past it."

I felt that way soon after I started floating. I wanted to go to the edge and discover what's out there. I wanted to feel deeper levels of connection, understanding, and contentment, all of which happen effortlessly in a float tank.

Spiritual exploration means different things to all of us. But I've found that regardless of your leanings, the tank has a profound ability to help you enter that spiritual realm.

Think about all the ways you feel limited by your

human, biological existence rather than something deeper. Every day you put on clothes, and you feel the fabric touch your skin. You go out in the bright sun and have to squint your eyes from the brightness. Or you hear traffic noise, dogs barking, or people talking. All these physical elements create a constant stream of sensory input reminding you that you are a body, you are a person, and you are a human being. You are working, living, striving, and surviving in a physical realm. This is your life every day.

The amazing thing is the tank is designed to remove all the sensory input that makes you feel so human all the time. It blocks out all of the light, so you can't see. It gets rid of physical touch with skin-temperature salt water that makes you float with a feeling of zero gravity. It's a silent environment with nothing to hear. Throw in nothing to smell or taste and you have pretty much nothing to remind you of your humanness. How powerful is that?

In a float tank, you leave behind the trappings of human existence and you are a spirit having a spiritual experience. For some, this experience involves thinking on deeper topics or issues in life. For others, it's feeling the connection between themselves and the universe with nothing in the way. Or maybe it's the feeling of bliss with nothing to do, except to be. For most, it's an experience for which they don't have words. What is spiritual exploration for you?

For me, spiritual exploration is getting closer to what I call "great spirit." Some might call it God, others might call it higher consciousness. Regardless, I want to feel more connected and more in line with my purpose. I think we all feel like we're on a journey with a much deeper meaning than everyday life may present. We all have been through so many trials, tribulations, and challenges, and we want to think there is meaning to it, at least I do. For me, spiritual floating is feeling at peace, in line, and with purpose.

Without going into the details of my spiritual adventures, I will say I've had some amazing breakthroughs in the tank. I've had moments of pure bliss where I feel like I'm pulsing with joy, like a feeling of ecstasy that I had only previously felt while actually taking the drug ecstasy. In fact, one of the reasons floating appealed so much to me is that over a decade ago I had some amazing highs on drugs like ecstasy, marijuana, and mushrooms, but the drugs really made my life unmanageable. When people told me I could reach these highs in the tank, and that I'd remember all of the experience, I was very intrigued.

Having tried both, I will say you can reach some pretty intense states naturally in the tank, not quite a drug state but very close. The benefit of the tank of course is that you stay in control, comfortable, and you can leave whenever you want.

I've also had moments of total understanding where a challenging issue finally made more sense. I've spent many a float thinking about deep long-term issues in my life, and I've left feeling more at peace with them. At one time I was ashamed of taking medication, seeing a counselor, or having problems the world could see. But with the help of floating, I've come to peace with them. Writing this book is a big testament to my self-acceptance. I'm proud to feel totally comfortable telling my story to the world. I don't believe I would have achieved this level of self-acceptance without floating.

The last spiritual breakthrough I'll tell you about is one of purpose. I believe we are all connected, which many people do. But I actually believe there is more than just a natural physical connection. I believe there is a universe of divine intelligence reaching and striving towards some ultimate evolution. I feel like when my mind is quieted in a tank, I am receiving the connection more clearly, as if ideas are hitting me faster and harder.

The ideas are bigger and bolder than what I would have come up with on my own. It's like my antennae are up and my barriers are down. The universe is speaking to me and wants to evolve through me. There are more than just my ideas in the tank. I'm receiving the desires of the universe. It's very inspiring to feel like you're connected to a higher purpose, rather than just a human wanting your way. Like you're wanting what the universe wants. There is great power in alignment with what the universe wants.

I know this all gets pretty heavy and deep. But I want you to know that whatever spiritual path you're on, or thoughts you may have about this crazy thing we call life, they will be amplified and purified in a float tank. How could they not be? Everything that distracts you from your spiritual self is eliminated. There has never been an environment like this in human history allowing you to be so effortlessly non-human. To set yourself free in a non-physical realm where the only limitations are time. To experience yourself with no barriers or outside factors. It's something that cannot be explained easily and is best experienced for yourself.

WHERE TO FLOAT

Now that you know you want to float and you understand more about what it may do for you, where do you go?

Recently, the Floatation Tank Association estimated that there are more than 200 float centers in the United States. This number is rising rapidly with more centers planned in cities large and small.

Many people have a float center conveniently located near their homes. If that's the case for you, I strongly recommend that you book a time and try it. The experienced technicians can guide you and help you get the most from your first—or fiftieth—float.

Here are some tips from Ashkahn Jahromi, co-owner of Float On in Portland, Oregon, on choosing a good float center:

- The environment should be clean and well-maintained—whether it's in a storefront or a private home.
- The water should be clear and a comfortable temperature.

*For more float tank locations, visit
FloatationLocations.com

- Noise should be kept at a minimum.
- If floating is only one of many options offered at a spa, be sure the person working is very familiar with floating and knows what they're doing.
- Owners or technicians who float themselves are always good indicators.

If you've floated before or already know it's something you want to do regularly, you might look into buying a tank for home use. This option is great for people who want to float multiple times a week or who don't have float centers near their homes.

Any tank can be used in the home. But the obstacles for most people are tank cost, shipping cost, and installation. Some of the bigger commercial tanks will be very difficult to physically get into your house. Also, their size and weight make shipping expensive. There are however affordable float tanks that are easier to ship and can be broken down for easier installation. Here are my top three for home use:

1. The Zen Float Tent offers the most affordable in-home option that starts under $2,000. It's like no other float tank on the market because it's made of flexible materials that can be packed and shipped in small boxes anywhere in the world.

2. The Escape Pod comes in at just about $8,000 for a complete float tank. It's a rigid traditional tank that looks great. It ships broken down in a small freight shipment. A great option for the home.

3. Last but not least, the Samadhi Tank is the original float tank created by Glenn and Lee Perry, who

were researchers with John Lilly. These tanks are tried and true, and they come in at about $12,000. The Samadhi is also a traditional tank design making it easy to move into a home and assemble.

Between these three options you will surely be able to find a tank just right for your home and your float habit.

I need to mention, having a tank in your home has huge benefits but it doesn't always make financial sense. I made a quick cost calculator I can send you to see if home floating is right for you. Email me and I'll send it to you.*

HOW OFTEN TO FLOAT

My float practice has become such a huge part of my life that I can't imagine my days without it. But I only feel that way now because in the beginning I started practicing more than just floating—I practiced a state of being.

I believe our life gives us more of what our state is. If you're a calm, peaceful person, your life will tend towards peace and tranquility. If you're a high-stress dramatic person, your life will attract stressful, dramatic situations and people. We very much get back in life the state we practice.

Early on when I began floating, I remember seeing my life change around me. I went from a state of chasing and addictive behavior to a state of calm and centeredness. It didn't happen overnight. I practiced a new state of being one float at a time.

*Email me at thefloattankcure@gmail.com

Today, that state of being has spread into all areas of my life, including my work, relationships, and self-esteem. I've found that I can remember and access that state anytime.

Whether you're floating to address anxiety and depression, improve athletic performance or decrease pain, or if you just want to expand your spiritual awareness, the most important aspect of the practice is actually to practice.

How often and how long you float is an individual choice. Each person gets something different from floating.

"You can describe it day in and day out," Ashkahn says, "but ultimately it's such a personal experience. It's such a unique experience, not only to each person but every float is totally unique. It's been years now, and I still hop in and have no idea what to expect in a certain sense. I'm like, okay, what is this float going to be like?

"Ultimately there's really no replacement for just hopping in a float tank and trying it. And trying it frequently. It's one of those things that doesn't quite reveal itself to you all the time through just a single float. Some of the best experiences we see people have are when they float once or twice a week, every week for a few weeks."

Once in the tank, everyone does what feels natural. Some people enjoy listening to music for a set amount of time—or nature sounds or chimes. Others like to stretch their muscles until they feel more relaxed and can enjoy the remainder of their float in peace.

Time of day also varies. A lot of people enjoy floating at night to inspire restful sleep, but for others, floating right before bedtime is too mentally stimulating. Afternoon floats in place of a nap can be restorative. And of course, a morning float is my favorite for extending that state between waking and dreaming.

Depending on your goals, I've developed a few suggested floating routines that you might try. But I strongly encourage you to use these simply as starting points. Don't be afraid to experiment with what works for your natural rhythms and daily habits.

I must open this section by emphasizing that I am not a doctor. I am not a health care professional. All of what you are about to read is my opinion from what I've seen, heard, and experienced. Please consult your health care professional before making any decisions with floating.

INTAKE OVERLOAD AND STRESS ROUTINE

If you're suffering from intake overload it's usually in a pattern following your work week. My recommendation would be to start your week off on the right foot with a float. Maybe that's a Sunday night for you to prepare for Monday morning or maybe you have the time to do an early morning float before work.

I'm currently floating Monday mornings, and it gives me a chance to think through my week, then quit thinking and get in a state of float. This sets the tone for my whole week. I get focused and feeling good first thing.

Watch how your mood pours into your week. It's pretty incredible.

If you're looking to get even more advanced, I would recommend wrapping up your overloaded work week with a float on a Friday. I also do this and have found it's the quickest way to settle down and turn my brain down a notch. When you first hop in, you'll also have the chance to go through your week, the wins, the losses, and prepare for the weekend.

I would also recommend floating with preparation in mind. If you know you have a particularly stressful week approaching, plan a float right in the middle. This will serve to break up the intensity so the stress doesn't compound day after day. If you have an event coming up that's going to stress you out, float before the event and use visualization to see yourself performing well. I float the day before I'm supposed to speak, and I feel so much calmer and more prepared. I knock down my stress level, and it makes a big difference.

In my experience, floating once a week will dramatically reduce overload and stress. But you've got to maintain the habit. You're better off going once a week and feeling like it's a bonus than not floating for a few weeks and crashing again. If you can get a float in twice a week, I doubt you'll even recognize your stress levels in a matter of weeks.

ANXIETY ROUTINE

This is my specialty because at one time my anxiety was spiraling out of control. If you want to reduce anxiety, you're going to need to float as often as possible. For daily anxiety, I highly recommend that you also meditate daily, even ten minutes a day will help a lot. Guided meditations by people like Karin Leonard are a great way to begin. Trust me, I know.

You can start with a weekly float habit and a daily meditation. Anxiety creeps up just when you're feeling good, so don't stop maintaining. Depression seems to move in like a slow thunderstorm, but anxiety can appear out of nowhere. So don't let up and don't get too confident that you're "fixed." Just find a float habit that you can stick to and do it.

If you have trouble floating weekly, at least get in the habit of daily meditation. I can't stress this enough. It works like magic, and if you find yourself graduating to floating, even better.

DEPRESSION ROUTINE

Depression is a creeping soul killer. It comes on slow and steady, and the next thing you know you can't even find the strength to push on anymore. Sometimes you don't even recognize your own life. Everything is dark and sad and hopeless. I know the feeling, I've been through it. Since depression usually doesn't link to an event or situation, this routine is all about habit and frequency.

First things first, you need to float as often as possible. I would shoot for weekly to start. My weekly habits are very powerful at keeping me happy. I float a couple times a week, I go to the gym a couple times a week, and I do something fun with friends once a week. These are the things that keep me happy and sane. That is why

I recommend doing a weekly float.

I understand this routine might not be doable for some people, but I would say do it as often as you can. Maybe that's every few weeks or monthly. Work in the floats when you can and try to build up the frequency as you see the benefits taking hold.

PAIN RELIEF ROUTINE

If you're floating to relieve pain, you are probably in one of two camps: healing from an injury or living with diagnosed, chronic pain.

For healing after an injury or surgical procedure, I usually recommend that people float as needed. Now you may want to add some maintenance floats weekly if you're the type that really pushes yourself and may sustain frequent strains. Otherwise, just float when it's obvious you need it. A float center near you is the perfect fit.

Chronic pain requires a more aggressive approach. The more time in the tank the better. Start by establishing a maintenance routine, whether that's weekly or even biweekly if that's what you can manage. Then add floats as you can do them.

The cost of a float center might be prohibitive for chronic pain sufferers who want multiple floats per week. If the average cost of a float is $50, it adds up fast. This would be a perfect situation to get a float tank in your home. When you divide the cost over twelve months, you might end up saving money and floating more often. Not to mention, being able to hop in the tank when your pain is acute is priceless.

ATHLETIC PERFORMANCE ROUTINE

I have talked to many marathon runners who say floating after a race is the quickest way to heal. UFC fighters and cross-fit trainers also recommend the practice for recovering from extreme or high-level sports. I have personally pushed myself very hard at the gym and felt so sore I couldn't even walk up my stairs. These are the types of situations when float tanks really speed up recovery. So aim for regular post-workout or event floats.

If you push yourself all the time in your sport, you might need an in-home tank as part of your training strategy. Whatever the case, you should probably shoot for a float every time you need to speed up healing, and that will depend on how often you're doing your thing.

A FINAL WORD ON CREATING A HABIT

I am an achievement junkie. I've studied success habits and personal growth strategies for years. I've seen the power of a habit over a flash of good intention countless times. Some people start a hobby and buy all the gear, only to never actually do the hobby. Some people go to the gym every day in January only to cancel their membership in February. And others have amazing ideas and work hard for a week only to lose interest a couple weeks later. This is the dysfunction I see that will push its way into your floating habit.

"START SMALL, STAY CONSISTENT, AND LET

THE SUCCESS FUEL YOUR FREQUENCY."

My recommendation: Shoot for a strong habit of floating even if it's only once a month. Stick to it until it's part of your routine, and you're comfortable with it. Don't let up until it's part of your regular life. Even with a slow, monthly habit you will start to see results and you will likely notice your life begin to improve.

This crucial first success is what will fuel a more frequent float habit and will give you the best odds of gaining all the benefits of floating.

But here's what I *don't* want you to do: Rush off to a float center, float every day at the expense of your wallet, time, and other habits that are equally as important, and create severe unbalance in your life. That unbalance will force you back out of floating as quickly as you got in.

Start small, stay consistent, and let the success fuel your frequency. This same motto applies to all positive habits you are trying to acquire. I learned the value of habits from a book called *The Compound Effect* by my mentor Darren Hardy. No, I don't get any kickbacks for this mention, and at the time of writing this he has no idea I'm even recommending it. The reason I am though, is habits are powerful, and I think everyone should learn how to create them. They will improve your life in so many ways, little by little, day by day.

THE FLOAT CURE

These last few years have been the most productive breakthrough years of my life. Mental focus, control, and overall calm have been essential to it all. Not only have I enjoyed the direct benefits of these improvements, but I've also been able to lay the foundation for new adventures. I've been in constant pursuit of learning, growing, and pushing my comfort zone. With all of this combined, my life has been a rocket ship.

And the single greatest thing about my journey so far is that I have the privilege of taking you along with me.

Floating truly is a therapeutic, enjoyable, and relaxing experience that everyone should be having on a regular basis. I hope this book will act as a gateway to floating for you. There are so many reasons to try floating, and it's becoming more and more convenient to do so. I urge you to call a float center near you and make your first appointment.

Don't forget to try floating at least three times before you decide what it is to you. Also, even though I've discussed many possibilities of what can happen in a tank, I urge you to have no expectations. Whatever happens, happens. You will have your best floats when they unfold naturally without thought or direction.

There's nothing more valuable than a healthy, happy mind and body. The best stuff in life rarely pays dividends up front. Most of the return happens in the long term. I hope this book has inspired you to invest in your long-term health and happiness. As you become more peaceful, more joyful, and more positive, that goodness will spread to others around you. When we float and create calm in our own lives, we create a ripple effect to everyone around us.

Thank you for hopping in the tank with me and starting a ripple effect of your own.

Happy Floating!

I hope you enjoyed The Float Tank Cure, and if you haven't already, I hope you book a float at your local center to try this amazing therapy out for yourself. It truly is life changing. If I could ask for one favor it would be this. Can I get your review?

With every review this book will become more credible, and the more credible it becomes the more new people will stumble onto it while book shopping. Your review will literally help spread the word of floating to more people, and that has always been my #1 goal.

So I would love your help and I'm kindly asking for your honest review now. If you don't mind.

Thank you.

-Shane

(FYI: you can always review the book on Amazon, even if you didn't purchase it there)

THE FLOAT
TANK CURE

by
SHANE STOTT

ACKNOWLEDGEMENTS

I want to first off thank my wife, Jamie, for putting up with me through everything I take on. She is the one who catches me when I crash and picks me up when I fall. I have a habit of taking on too much all the time, and she is the reason I can keep going. Thanks, babe, for the support.

Second, I want to thank my editor, Amy Anderson, who takes all of my float ramblings, ideas, thoughts, and interviews, and crafts them into a nice, polished book. I promise you, this book wouldn't be half as good without her. Thank you, Amy, you're amazing.

Third, I want to thank William Hill for reaching out to me to be a part of this grand idea to make floating accessible to the world. It was such a moment of alignment for my life. Thank you, my dear friend.

Fourth, thank you to Darren Hardy for showing me that I should write a book and that I have a gift to offer people. As it turns out, it's been very enjoyable writing my entire story, and the gift truly was mine. So thank you, Darren, for the eye opener.

Fifth, Stephen Woessner, for pushing me to just write the book already and quit waiting! Thank you, Stephen, for the kick in the butt when I needed it. You make all this stuff look easy. You are the inspiration that got this book started.

Sixth, I really want to thank my book launch crew who helped me make everything happen. Jennifer Maffei for all the scheduling, planning, and coordinating that allowed the book and interviews to come together quickly. Jaymie Tarshis for being my right hand through the endless to-do list of launching a book—she is the reason this book happened on time and smoothly. Jason Malaska for all the help getting to Amazon and making the book look nice in any format. Ryan Holiday for the book launch strategy—he truly is the king of book launches.

Last but not least, I want to thank my grandpa, Brent, who really is like a father to me. He's my role model in life and the reason I'm the man I am today. Thanks, grandpa.

IF YOU EMAIL ME AT

thefloattankcure@gmail.com

I WILL SEND YOU:

1. THE JOE ROGAN FLOAT VIDEO THAT INSPIRED ME TO BUILD A FLOAT TANK

2. LINKS TO MY FAVORITE KARIN LEONARD GUIDED MEDITATIONS

3. A QUICK GUIDE TO FIND OUT IF FLOATING AT HOME IS RIGHT FOR YOU.

CITED SOURCES

1   Suedfeld, Peter and Borrie, Roderick A. "Health and Therapeutic Applications of Chamber and Flotation Restricted Environmental Stimulation Therapy REST - Psychology and Health" (*Psychology & Health,*, University of British Columbia, Department of Psychology, 1999) 545-566.

2   Harry Mills, Ph.D., Natalie Reiss, Ph.D., and Mark Dombeck, Ph.D., "Types of Stressors (Eustress Vs. Distress)," (https://www.mentalhelp.net/articles/types-of-stressors-eustress-vs-distress/ 2008).

3   Same as above

4   Same as above

5   R. Moran Griffin, "10 Fixable Stress-Related Health Problems," WebMD http://www.webmd.com/balance/stress-management/features/10-fixable-stress-related-health-problems

6   http://www.cdc.gov/ncbddd/adhd/data.html, "Attention-Deficit/Hyperactivity Disorder: Data & Statistics," Centers for Disease Control and Prevention.

7   U.S. Department of Health and Human Services, National Center for Complimentary and Integrative Health, a division of National Institute of Health, "The 2012 National Health Interview Survey: Use of Complimentary Health Approaches in the U.S.," https://nccih.nih.gov/research/statistics/NHIS/2012.

8   Suedfeld, Peter and Borrie, Roderick A., "Health and Therapeutic Applications of Chamber and Flotation Restricted Environmental Stimulation Therapy REST," (*Psychology & Health*, Department of Psychology, University of British Columbia 1999)

545-566.

9   J. W. Turner Jr and T. H. Fine, "Restricting Environmental Stimulation Influences Levels and Variability of Plasma Cortisol," (*Journal of Applied Physiology*, http://jap.physiology.org/content/70/5/2010 1991).

10   Fine, T. H., and J. W. Turner Jr. The Use of Restricted Environmental Stimulation Therapy (REST) in the Treatment of Essential Hypertension," (*First International Conference on REST and Self-regulation* 1985).

11   U.S. Department of Health and Human Services: Substance Abuse and Mental Health Services Administration, *The 2012 National Survey on Drug Use and Health (NSDUH): Mental Health Findings* http://www.samhsa.gov/data/sites/default/files/2k12MH_Findings/2k12MH_Findings/NSDUHmhfr2012.htm.

12   Anxiety and Depression Association of America, "Understanding the Facts of Anxiety Disorders and Depression Is the First Step." http://www.adaa.org/understanding-anxiety.

13   Same as above.

14   Same as above.

15   Anxiety and Depression Association of America, "Panic Disorder & Agoraphobia." http://www.adaa.org/understanding-anxiety/panic-disorder-agoraphobia.

16   Suedfeld, Peter and Borrie, Roderick A., "Health and Therapeutic Applications of Chamber and Flotation Restricted Environmental Stimulation Therapy REST," (*Psychology & Health*, Department of Psychology, University of British Columbia 1999) 545-566.

17   Anxiety and Depression Association of America, "Facts and Statistics." http://www.adaa.org/about-adaa/press-room/facts-statistics.

18   S.A. Bood, U. Sundequist, A. Kjellgren, G. Nordstrom, and T. Norlander, "Effects of Flotation-Restricted Environmental Stimulation Technique on Stress-Related Muscle Pain: What Makes the Difference in Therapy—Attention-Placebo or the Relaxation Response?"(*Pain Research & Management* 2005) 201-9.

19   Anxiety and Depression Association of America, "Post-traumatic Stress Disorder." http://www.adaa.org/understanding-anxiety/posttraumatic-stress-disorder-ptsd.

20   U.S. Department of Health and Human Services, National Institutes of Health, "Pain Management." http://report.nih.gov/nihfactsheets/ViewFactSheet.aspx?csid=57.

21   Harvard Medical School: Harvard Health Publications, "12 Things You Should Know About Pain Relievers." http://www.health.harvard.edu/pain/12-things-you-should-know-about-pain-relievers.

22   Mayo Clinic, "Antidepressants: Another Weapon Against Chronic Pain." http://www.mayoclinic.org/pain-medications/art-20045647.

23   Substance Abuse and Mental Health Services: "Types of Commonly Misused or Abused Drugs." http://www.samhsa.gov/prescription-drug-misuse-abuse/types.

24   Same as above

25   S.A. Bood, U. Sundequist, A. Kjellgren, G. Nordstrom, and T. Norlander , "Effects of Flotation-Restricted Environmental Stimulation Technique on Stress-Related Muscle Pain: What Makes the Difference in Therapy--Attention-Placebo or the Relaxation

Response?". (*Pain Research & Management* 2005) 201-9.

26   Institute of Medicine Report from the Committee on Advancing Pain Research, Care, and Education: *Relieving Pain in America: A Blueprint for Transforming Prevention, Care, Education and Research.* (The National Academies Press 2011).

27   Turner Jr, John, et al. "Effects of Flotation REST on Range of Motion, Grip Strength and Pain in Rheumatoid Arthritics." *Clinical and Experimental Restricted Environmental Stimulation.* Springer New York, 1993. 297-306.

28   Rzewnicki, Randy, et al. "REST for muscle contraction headaches: A comparison of two REST environments combined with progressive muscle relaxation training." *Restricted Environmental Stimulation.* Springer New York, 1990. 174-183.

29   Fine, Thomas H., and John W. Turner Jr. "Rest-assisted relaxation and chronic pain." *Health and clinical psychology* 4 (1985): 511-518.

30   R. Borrie, T. Russell, and S. Schneider , "The Effects of Flotation REST on the Symptoms of Fibromyalgia,". Presented at April 21 at Float Summit 2012 in Gothenburg, Sweden.

31   Nica[1], Adriana Sarah, Adela Caramoci, Mirela Vasilescu, Anca Mirela Ionescu, Denis Paduraru, and Virgil Mazilu. "Magnesium Supplementation in Top Athletes-Effects and Recommendations." Medicina Sportiva 11, no. 1 (2015): 2482-2494.

32   *The Washington Times* "Float Spa Fans Say Isolation Tanks Buoy Bodies and Minds." http://www.washingtontimes.com/news/2015/jun/9/float-spa-fans-say-isolation-tanks-buoy-bodies-and/?page=all.

33   Roure, R., et al. (1998). Autonomic Nervous System Responses Correlate with Mental Rehearsal in Volleyball Training. *Journal of Applied Physiology*, 78(2), 99-108.

34   Suedfeld, Peter, and Geraldine Schwartz. "Restricted Environmental Stimulation Therapy (REST) as a Treatment for Autistic Children." *Journal of Developmental & Behavioral Pediatrics* 4.3 (1983): 196-201.

35   Suedfeld, Peter and Borrie, Roderick A., "Health and Therapeutic Applications of Chamber and Flotation Restricted Environmental Stimulation Therapy REST," *Psychology & Health*, Vol.14, Iss.3, 1999, Pp 545-566., Department of Psychology, University of British Columbia.

36   Peter Suedfeld PhD, "Retricted Environmental Stimulation Therapy of Smoking: A Parametric Study", Department of Psychology 2002, University of British Columbia, Vancouver, B.C.

THE FLOAT
TANK CURE

FREE YOURSELF FROM STRESS, ANXIETY, AND PAIN THE NATURAL WAY

by
SHANE STOTT